You Can Discover the Many Benefits of a Healthy, Relaxed, Stress-Free Life.

Give yourself a break. You can meet every challenge, overcome everyday problems. You can put the headaches and backaches behind you. You can eat well, sleep better, and add new vitality to your family life, social life and career. The key is stress management, and with this book you can enjoy a life full of excitement and challenge while you learn how to deal with and neutralize the pressures and anxieties that stand in your way.

All it takes is a sound, balanced diet, a program of simple aerobic exercises—swimming, dancing, cycling or whatever you choose—and an easy-to-master, soothing routine of relaxation and revitalization.

Give yourself a break. Give yourself...

**The Alive & Well®
Stress Book**

QUANTITY PURCHASES

ALIVE
&
WELL®
STRESS
BOOK

by Marc Leepson

BANTAM BOOKS
TORONTO • NEW YORK • LONDON • SYDNEY • AUCKLAND

For Janna

ALIVE & WELL® STRESS BOOK

A Bantam Book / August 1984

ALIVE AND WELL® and its letter device are registered trademarks of Bristol-Myers Company. Registered in U.S. Patent and Trademark Office and elsewhere.

Charts by Paul Woolner
Front cover photograph courtesy of Photofile

ISBN 0-553-24366-7

Published simultaneously in the United States and Canada

Bantam Books are published by Bantam Books, Inc. Its trademark, consisting of the words "Bantam Books" and the portrayal of a rooster, is Registered in U.S. Patent and Trademark Office and in other countries. Marca Registrada. Bantam Books, Inc., 666 Fifth Avenue, New York, New York 10103.

PRINTED IN THE UNITED STATES OF AMERICA

H   0 9 8 7 6 5 4 3 2 1

Contents

Stress Producers

1 / Test Yourself

Here's a quick way to find out right off the bat whether you're suffering from stress. The first thing to remember is that no one is immune from stress. Births and deaths, marriages and divorces, and hirings and firings, all bring with them a healthy—or not-so-healthy—dose of stress.

Doctors who specialize in treating stress-related disorders usually subject their patients to long, detailed written examinations to determine the level of stress in their daily lives. But in the late 1960s, psychiatrists Thomas Holmes and Richard H. Rahe developed a chart that provides an accurate gauge of the everyday life events that cause stress.

Dr. Holmes, of the University of Washington's School of Medicine, has studied the physical and psychological implications involved in changes in life. After examining the details of the lives of more than 5,000 patients, Dr. Holmes concluded that certain events were associated with the onset of various illnesses, from skin eruptions to tuberculosis. Some of the life events that seemed to precipitate illnesses were negative: being fired from a job, getting divorced, and so on. Other disease-producing events, according to Dr. Holmes, were not necessarily unpleasant: marriage, the birth of a child, assuming a new job.

The common denominator in these life events was the change itself. And with the vast changes involved in today's fast-paced life-styles, those who expend all their energy trying to cope with change can exhaust their bodily defenses, and run an increased risk of being stricken with a stress-related physical disease.

Dr. Holmes uses the analogy of an overburdened computer programmed with more information than it is designed to handle. When the computer's circuits become overloaded with information, it breaks down. Coping with change can weaken a human being's "circuits" to the point where one of them gives out and we develop an illness.

To find out if events in your life are ganging up on you and increasing your risk of contracting major stress-related illnesses, read through the following chart developed by Dr. Holmes and his colleague, Dr. Richard H. Rahe. If, in the past 12 months, you have experienced any of the life events listed in the first column, note their values and total the numbers.

Death of spouse	100
Divorce	73
Marital separation	65
Jail term	63
Death of close family member	63
Personal injury or illness	53
Marriage	50
Fired at work	47
Marital reconciliation	45
Retirement	45
Change in health of family member	44
Pregnancy	40
Sex difficulties	39
Gain of new family member	39
Business readjustment	39
Change in financial state	38

Death of close friend	37
Change to different line of work	36
Change in number of arguments with spouse	35
Mortgage over $10,000	31
Foreclosure of mortgage or loan	30
Change in responsibilities at work	29
Son or daughter leaving home	29
Trouble with in-laws	29
Outstanding personal achievement	28
Wife or husband begins or ends work	26
Begin or end of school	26
Change in living conditions	25
Revision of personal habits	24
Trouble with boss	23
Change in work hours or conditions	20
Change in residence	20
Change in schools	20
Change in recreation	19
Change in religious activities	18
Change in social activities	18
Mortgage or loan less than $10,000	17
Change in sleeping habits	16
Change in number of family get-togethers	15
Change in eating habits	15
Vacation	13
Christmas	12
Minor violations of the law	11[1]

If your score is from 0 to 149, you are in the "low" stress category. You really don't have much to worry about, although you still have a 30-percent chance of experiencing what psychiatrists call a stress-related health change. This includes not only serious illnesses, but also injuries, surgical operations, and psychological problems.

Your chances of having a moderate stress-related health change rise to 50 percent if you scored between 150 and

300 points. The chance then jumps to 80 percent if you scored over 300. This is called major life stress.

Now that you've learned what stress category you are in—low, moderate, or major—here's a way to find out if you are able to handle that stress.

The following chart contains 45 questions, including 6 for women only. Check in the appropriate column whether you experience each symptom rarely or often. Once you've completed the chart and gone over your answers, it should become obvious to you if you're able to control your stress.

	RARELY	OFTEN
1. Do you feel irritable, hyperactive, or depressed?		
2. Do you feel your heart pounding extra hard?		
3. Do you have heartburn?		
4. Do you breathe rapidly?		
5. Is your throat and/or mouth excessively dry?		
6. Do you tremble or have nervous tics?		
7. Do you break out in nervous, high-pitched laughter?		
8. Do your hands shake?		
9. Do you stutter?		
10. Do you suffer from dizziness?		
11. Do you have diarrhea?		
12. Do you have severe indigestion?		

RARELY   OFTEN

13. Are your hands and feet cold?
14. Do you sweat profusely?
15. Do you frequently need to urinate?
16. Do you suffer from migraine headaches?
17. Do you have nightmares?
18. Do you have insomnia?
19. Do you have a lot of trouble getting out of bed in the morning?
20. Are you able to concentrate on your daily tasks?
21. Are you bored?
22. Does your body in general just feel weak?
23. Do you grind your teeth?
24. Do you eat to excess?
25. Do you skip meals or eat very small amounts of food at mealtime?
26. Do you drink alcohol heavily?
27. Do you use prescription drugs to excess?
28. Do you use illicit drugs— marijuana or cocaine—to excess?
29. Do you smoke cigarettes heavily?
30. Do you feel trapped by life?
31. Do you get angry easily?

RARELY   OFTEN

32. Are you accident-prone?
33. Do you hate waiting in line?
34. Is your commute to work filled with nervous tension?
35. Are you very competitive at work and at play?
36. Do you lose your temper when something unexpected happens?
37. Do you do things impulsively?
38. Do you feel anxious for no apparent reason?
39. Do you seem to be doing two things at once, without ever getting anything done?

FOR WOMEN ONLY

40. Do you have intense premenstrual pain?
41. Is your menstrual cycle irregular?
42. Do you depend on your husband for nearly everything?
43. Are you obsessed with your personal appearance?
44. Do you depend on your children to make you happy?
45. Do you feel the need to depend on your sexuality to make friends?

If you checked often on 7 or more of these questions, it's very possible that your body and mind are trying to tell you something:, Stress is eating at you, and you should do something about it before things get worse.

The next chapter tells you exactly what this bogeyman called stress is; how some stress actually is good for you; and how stress affects both men and women in the same manner.

---

1. T. H. Holmes and R. H. Rahe, *Journal of Psychosomatic Research* XI (1967).

2 / Definition of Stress Differences Between Positive and Negative Stress

To a physicist, stress is the capacity of a structure to withstand pressure exerted upon it. To a biologist, stress is anything that threatens to adversely affect an organism. To most laymen, stress is undesirable pressure from life that brings discomfort, tension, worry, and frustration.

But to psychologists, stress is something different. In psychology, stress does *not* refer to outside pressure that affects behavior, but to the body's *response* to these pressures. Stress, in fact, is not necessarily bad. It serves useful functions; it prepares you to meet a threat or to perform certain physical tasks.

Dr. Hans Selye, the Vienna-born endocrinologist, and the world's leading expert on stress in his classic book, *The Stress of Life,* provided several examples of what stress is *not.*

Stress is not, Dr. Selye claims, merely nervous tension because lower animals and plants—organisms that do not have nervous systems—experience stress. And stress can be produced in humans even when we are unconscious.

Stress is not the emergency discharge of adrenaline,

according to Dr. Selye, because even though adrenaline and stress are indirectly linked, stress is not the only reason why the body produces adrenaline.

Stress is not merely something that causes direct damage. A passionate kiss, Dr. Selye points out, can cause considerable stress, but probably won't cause any damage.

Stress is not something that causes the body to go into an alarm reaction because the *stressor* (the event that triggers stress) does that, not stress itself.

Lastly, stress cannot—and should not—be avoided. We are all under some form of stress at all times, even while asleep.

What then is stress? Dr. Selye provides this definition. "Stress is the state manifested by a specific syndrome which consists of all the nonspecifically induced changes within a biologic system."[1] That sounds like a mouthful of medical-psychological jargon. But, simply put, Dr. Selye is saying that stress is a bodily state of being brought about by a specific series of biological events.

The reason that stress is "nonspecifically induced" is that while very specific changes happen in the body, these changes are caused by many different things. Dr. Selye explains that some stress responses result from any type of stimulus, from a kiss to a car accident. Dr. Selye avoids using the term, but essentially, we can simplify his definition by saying that stress is the *rate of wear and tear* on the body caused by the many and varied events that happen to us every moment of our lives.

In a 1977 interview, Dr. Selye put his definition in simple terms. He went on to say: "I define stress as the nonspecific response of the body to a demand."

> Stress is the state you are in, not the agent which produces it, which is called a stressor. Cold and heat, for example, are stressors. But, in man, with his highly developed central nervous system,

11

emotional stressors are the most frequent and the most important... The thing for the average person to remember is that all the demands that you make—whether on your brain or your liver or your muscles or your bones—cause stress.[2]

The Human Body's Response to Stress

Let's take a look at exactly what happens to the human body under stress. Dr. Selye divides the human response to stress—what is called the general adaptation syndrome—into three stages.

First, in the *alarm reaction* stage, the body is taken by surprise. You recognize stress, resistance to it temporarily fades, and the brain sends a message to the pituitary gland. This gland then produces a hormone which induces the adrenal glands to secrete substances including adrenaline. When this happens, your pulse begins to race and you may begin to perspire.

Then, in the *resistance stage*, the body begins to marshal its resources to fight back against the outside stressor. The production of adrenaline and other hormones is stepped up, and you are usually able to resist or adapt to whatever it is that is causing the stress.

Stage three is the *exhaustion* stage, in which prolonged stress causes the body to become depleted and resistance fails. This phase results in the wear and tear of the body we referred to earlier. In extreme cases, it can even lead to death.

The "Fight-or-Flight" Syndrome

Let's say you are walking down the street on your way to work one day. You decide to take a different route than the one you normally use. You turn a corner, and nearly run into a large, disheveled street bum. He looks at you, mumbles something about the economy, and begins following you, shouting at you, demanding money.

No matter how many times this happens to you, your body reacts in the same manner, and it reacts involuntarily. Your muscles tense. Your hearing becomes finely tuned. Your red blood cells rush throughout your body, carrying oxygen to the muscles and the brain. Your heart rate increases. Your blood pressure climbs. All your senses, in fact, heighten.

You are experiencing the fight-or-flight syndrome, something that has been a part of human beings for millennia. In this initial response of the body to an outside threat, the entire system becomes mobilized for action—either to escape the situation quickly (flight), or to be prepared to battle it out (fight).

When primitive man experienced fight-or-flight, the situation usually was a literal choice between fighting a dangerous beast or running full speed away from the danger. But for most of us today, the body goes into its fight-or-flight mode under very different circumstances.

The phone rings at three o'clock in the morning. A little child chasing a ball runs out in front of your car. The boss calls you into her office for an unexpected meeting. Your child brings home a note saying his history teacher wants to discuss something personally with you.

In these situations, your brain unwittingly activates the fight-or-flight alarm system, but—unlike our primitive ancestors—you will not have to do battle or flee. If you continually activate the system in situations that don't call for it, you are mobilizing these emergency resources without using them. You are putting more and more wear and tear upon your body.

The fight-or-flight set of responses is not always harmful. In fact, it can be beneficial. If you find yourself in a burning building, for example, you'll be very happy to discover that you can run faster and think quicker than you ever believed possible. Or in a not-quite-so-dramatic situation, picture yourself on your morning jog when you're feeling not quite up to par, and you're thinking of quitting. Then, all of a sudden, you round a corner and see the homestretch of your run coming up. The relief of seeing your goal in reachable distance should trigger the fight-or-flight response mechanisms and provide you with the ability to forge on and complete your run.

This brings up the point of the beneficial aspects of stress. Just as the fight-or-flight response can help you in times of need, so, too can stress. In fact, stress is a vital requirement of life. Without any stress at all, the human animal cannot survive. The body has to be continually challenged and stimulated to survive. Doctors say that those who don't have enough stress in their lives suffer from *hypostress*—as opposed to those who are under too much pressure and suffer from *hyperstress*. The problems associated with hypostress and hyperstress can be similar: high blood pressure, increased risk of heart disease, muscular problems, and so on.

The amount of stress that each of us needs varies depending on the individual. One way to see if you are suffering from too much or too little stress is to divide up your day into three levels: constructive stress, destructive stress, and deadly stress (see the following charts). If most of what happens to you during the day stays in the constructive level—a gentle awakening in the morning, a relaxing early-morning exercise period, a smooth, pleasant commute to work, a busy but constructive day, and a relaxing evening—you are living a full life, being bombarded by stressors, but those stressors are positive. They are giving your body the stimulus it needs, both mental and physical, to keep going.

If, on the other hand, your daily schedule is full of

stressors that put you constantly in the destructive category—or worse, the deadly level—then you are inviting serious problems, unless you discover how to mitigate the effects of stress.

For Women Only

Stress does not discriminate by sex. Everything we've noted about the effects of stress applies equally to men and women. But women face a set of potential problems with stress that men do not have to deal with. Some of these problems have to do with the biological differences between the sexes; some have to do with the roles that women play in today's society.

On the biological level, experts say that the phases in life for women that bring with them the most stress-prone moments are puberty, motherhood, and menopause. Women who undertake the traditional roles of wife, homemaker, and mother do not have to be told how these roles can bring with them tensions and stresses in marriage and family rearing.

But today, with more and more women either forswearing the traditional role of wife and mother, or trying to combine that role with a career, the opportunities for stress-induced problems have increased drastically.

On the job, women face the same pressure their male counterparts are exposed to. But many women feel the need to try to strive harder than men in order to succeed. This can lead to all the stress-induced problems that men face—as they try to climb the ladder of success in the business world.

Since the number of single women raising families alone far outstrips the number of single male parents, these women also face a disproportionate share of stress both at work and at home. They feel the pressure to excel at work, to excel in extracurricular activities, as well as to excel in child rearing. Assuming the role of "supermother" carries with it a host of potential problems in the area of stress management.

Stress in Your Daily Routine

The following charts illustrate how your daily routine affects the level of stress you are under. These charts measure your activities from the time you awake until bedtime, and their contribution to what we call constructive, destructive, or deadly stress.

Two charts are filled in and the third is blank. We provide examples on the first two, and leave one for you to use on a typical day of your own.

The first chart follows a 35-year-old working mother of two school-age children through a typical workday. On this day, the woman sleeps through her alarm clock at 6:30 and doesn't get up unil 7:15. She's now 45 minutes late, and cannot prepare a hot breakfast for herself and the children. Nor can she properly oversee the kids' grooming and other preparations for school. Since she barely has time to fix the kids' lunches, this means skipping breakfast herself. This person's stress level is already in the destructive range before she even leaves the house.

The woman manages to get the kids to school on time, but is forced to hurry on to work to avoid being late. There is a big traffic jam on the way to the office, and by the time the woman gets to work, she feels tense. But she does make it on time. Clearly she is not under constructive stress levels.

By 10:00, our beleaguered friend has taken two aspirins because of a headache, and is fixing herself a second cup of coffee. She gulps down her coffee in a hurry with a sweet roll on the way to a hastily called staff meeting.

Definition of Stress Differences

Her computations on a statistical report contained two crucial errors and the boss scolds her during the meeting. She is told to redo the entire report, and the shipping department has to work several hours of overtime that night. Lunch consists of a tunafish sandwich, potato chips, and a soft drink eaten at her desk while she redoes the report. The report takes hours longer than she expected; she's forced to work overtime and has to make arrangements for a baby-sitter to take care of the children until she arrives home at 7:30. She fixes dinner for the children, and—totally exhausted—falls asleep in front of the TV set during the 11:00-news.

The second chart represents the day of a 40-year-old account representative and mother of two young teenagers. This woman awakes at 6:00, skips her usual exercise routine, and manages to get her two children to her sister's house and herself to the airport an hour early for an 8:30-flight. She has a cup of coffee and a bowl of cereal in the airport restaurant before boarding her plane.

The plane is held up because of bad weather, and lands 45 minutes late. She has to rush out of the airport, grab a taxi, and hurry to get to her appointment on time. The session goes very well; she lands a new account for the company, then celebrates with a drink with the client afterward. Her flight home is uneventful. She picks up the kids, takes them out for dinner, and spends a relaxing evening at home.

In looking at the two charts, we can see that both women had long and busy days, full of stressful situations. The first woman had a high level of stress that stayed mostly in the destructive level, but rose occasionally into the deadly level. Continuing this type of experience can lead to physical and emotional problems and can cause the woman's work performance to decline. This woman could be heading for problems that likely could include alcohol or drug abuse, depression, or emotional instability.

17

The second woman, on the other hand, has a day filled mostly with constructive stress, and if her life continues in this manner, she will not suffer from the problems potentially awaiting the first woman.

One way to get an indication of how your daily schedule fits into this model is to fill in the following blank chart. Pick a typical day and see how the stressors you encounter measure up.

The next chapter takes a look at the health consequences of a life-style that contains too much destructive stress.

1. Hans Selye, *The Stress of Life*, rev. ed. (New York: McGraw-Hill Book Company, 1978), p. 64.
2. Quoted in *U.S. News & World Report*, March 21, 1977, p. 51.

Chart 1

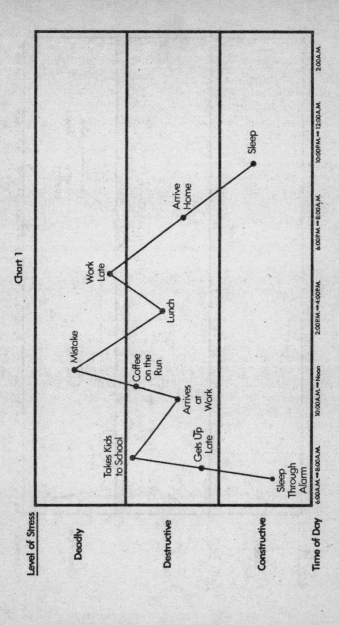

Level of Stress

Deadly

Destructive

Constructive

Time of Day

6:00 A.M. → 8:00 A.M.   10:00 A.M. → Noon   2:00 P.M. → 4:00 P.M.   6:00 P.M. → 8:00 A.M.   10:00 P.M. → 12:00 A.M.   2:00 A.M.

Mistake

Takes Kids to School

Coffee on the Run

Work Late

Arrives at Work

Lunch

Arrive Home

Gets Up Late

Sleep

Sleep Through Alarm

Chart 2

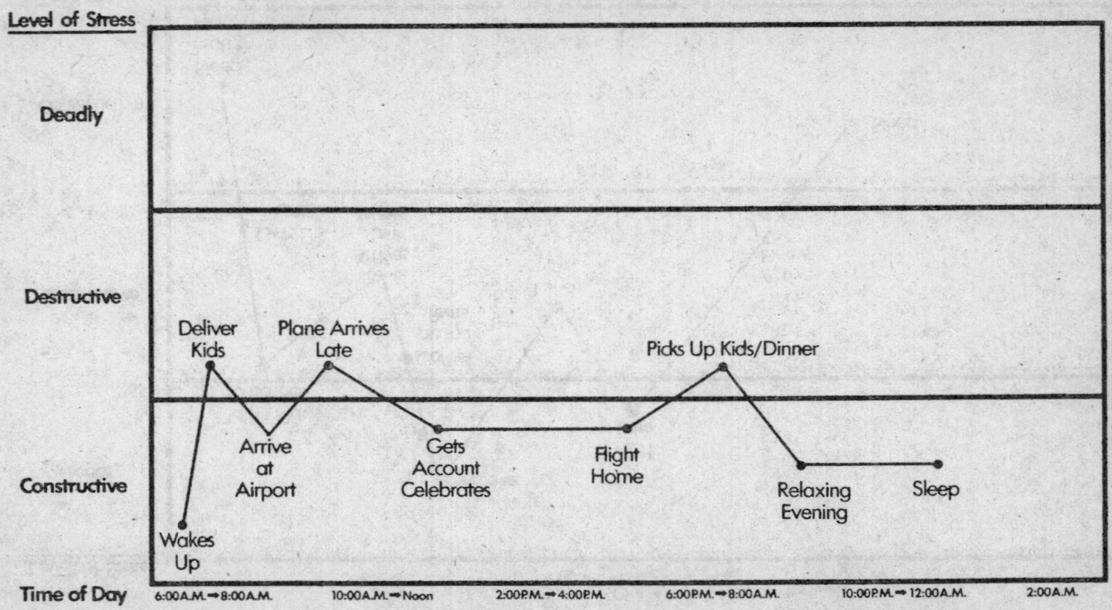

Level of Stress

Deadly

Destructive

Constructive

Time of Day

6:00A.M.→8:00A.M.   10:00A.M.→Noon   2:00P.M.→4:00P.M.   6:00P.M.→8:00A.M.   10:00P.M.→12:00A.M.   2:00A.M.

Wakes Up

Deliver Kids

Arrive at Airport

Plane Arrives Late

Gets Account Celebrates

Flight Home

Picks Up Kids/Dinner

Relaxing Evening

Sleep

Chart 3
(fill in your day)

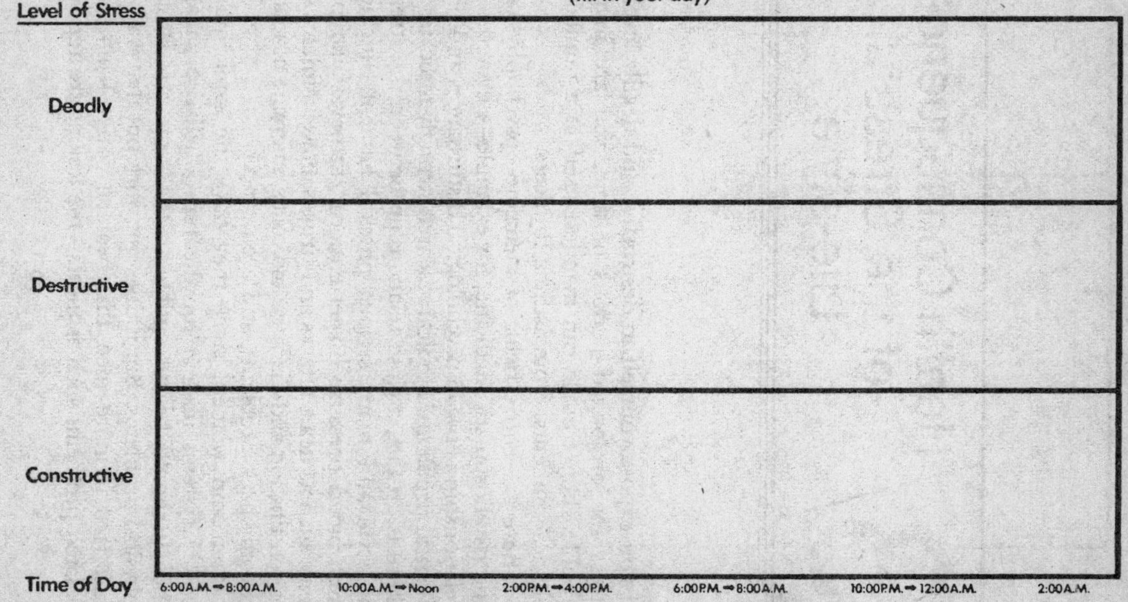

Level of Stress	6:00 A.M. → 8:00 A.M.	10:00 A.M. → Noon	2:00 P.M. → 4:00 P.M.	6:00 P.M. → 8:00 P.M.	10:00 P.M. → 12:00 A.M.	2:00 A.M.
Deadly						
Destructive						
Constructive						
Time of Day						

3 / Health Consequences of the Stressful Life-style

If you expose yourself to destructive and deadly levels of stress for prolonged periods of time, you are inviting trouble. This trouble can manifest itself in a number of physical ailments, from asthma to ulcers.

There are entire fields of medicine—psychophysiology and psychosomatic medicine, for example—devoted to the relationship between psychological disturbances and physiological problems. Medical research strongly indicates that there is, in fact, a close relationship between the stressful life-style and many serious physical ailments, including high blood pressure (hypertension), cardiovascular problems such as heart attacks and strokes, bowel ailments such as constipation and diarrhea and colitis, migraine headaches, chronic back problems, and even cancer.

Men and women, since they have the same internal bodily systems (except for the reproductive organs), in theory should be susceptible to the same stress-related physical problems. But it does not work out that way. The fact is that more men than women suffer from stress-related problems such as ulcers—the lesions created when the digestive juices eat away at the lining of the stomach—and cardiovascular ailments such as heart attacks.

Heart disease is the Number 1 killer in this country. More than 750,000 Americans die from it every year, according to the National Center for Health Statistics. There are many causes of heart disease. These include genetic predisposition, obesity, hypertension, high cholesterol levels in the blood, and cigarette smoking.

Another prime risk factor associated with heart disease is what has come to be known as the Type A personality. The term was coined by Drs. Meyer Friedman and Ray Rosenman in their 1974 books, *Type A Behavior and Your Heart.* A person with a Type A personality is someone who is very competitive and ambitious—two traits that bring with them much stress, but by themselves are not necessarily destructive. But Type As also suffer from "hurry-up sickness." That is, they are impatient and always fighting against the clock. This combination of traits produces a person who typically is a workaholic—someone who can't stop working day and night, weekdays and weekends.

The Type A person also cannot relax, and is usually extroverted and aggressive. This person is always in a hurry, and cannot abide waiting in line or being inconvenienced in any other way. He gets angry and hostile very easily but usually keeps this all-consuming aggressiveness and hostility directed inward, which can cause an extreme case of prolonged stress along with psychological and physical problems. In many cases, the unchecked Type A personality leads first to hypertension and then to some form of heart disease.

There are Type As for both sexes. But the statistics clearly indicate that more men than women are Type As. And more men than women suffer from hypertension and ulcers, the two most common stress-related physical ailments. This is not to say that women are immune from these problems. Obviously, they are not, and women should be concerned about them.

There are a number of stress-related physical ailments that affect women more than men. These include migraine headaches and muscle-related conditions such as pain in the shoulder and neck, and backaches. These aches often are caused when we unwittingly transfer the psychic tensions of our daily lives directly into our skeletal muscles—the muscles involved in movement and posture that are found all along the skeletal frame.

What happens is that stressful moments in life cause us to tense up certain muscles involuntarily, and these muscles contract partially. When someone is exposed to stressors for long periods of time, the muscles can contract into painful, hard knots. These can occur anywhere in the body. When the muscles in the head contract, they cause headaches.

There are many muscles in the head. Some of them are small, such as the tiny muscles that make our eyes blink. Some are very large, such as the frontalis muscles, which are located in the forehead.

When a biofeedback therapist (see p. 152) wants to measure the tension in a patient's muscles, he attaches a sensor to the frontalis muscles on the forehead. Measuring the tension in these muscles provides the best indicator of the amount of tension a person is holding in the upper body. When the frontalis muscle contracts for a prolonged period of time, a headache develops. Contractions occur when we frown, think heavily, knot our brows, or even squint.

A sure way to create tension in the facial muscles is by clenching your jaw. The important spot here is the temporomandibular joint (TMJ). You can feel this area by gritting your teeth, and putting your index finger on either side of your jaw at the point where your upper and lower jaws meet just below the ear. When you grit your teeth, you can feel the TMJ contract and bulge out. Prolonged contraction can cause pain throughout the head, jaw, and face.

A similar problem, called bruxism, occurs when you grit your teeth so that your upper and lower teeth surfaces come in contact with each other. Those suffering from bruxism often find themselves grinding their teeth in their sleep. They awake to excruciating pain in the teeth and jaws.

Most people who sit at a desk for most of the working day wind up putting tremendous tension into their trapezius muscles, the two large L-shaped muscles that extend from the base of the skull behind the ears down the back of the neck and outward along the tops of the shoulders. These long muscles often are the repository of a great deal of tension. This can result in pains in the neck and shoulder, and even headaches.

There are two basic types of headaches—muscular and vascular. The headaches we've just discussed all fall under the category of muscular headaches since they are caused by prolonged muscular tension. The other group, vascular headaches, includes one of the least understood physical ailments, the migraine.

Some persons feel that any severe headache is a migraine. But this is not the case because migraine headaches have a number of specific characteristics. For one thing, migraines are not caused by muscular tension. A migraine is considered a vascular headache because it's caused by dysfunction in the flow of blood to the head.

When the arteries carrying blood from the heart to the brain constrict and then swell, the result is the migraine headache. This pain usually affects only one side of the head, hence the meaning of the word *migraine*, from the Greek *hemikrania*, meaning "half of the skull."

Doctors do not know with certainty what causes migraine headaches. But they do know that a set of emotional factors often plays a role in the onset of migraines.

Many migraine sufferers are ultra-competitive, compulsive persons who are not easily satisfied. When such a migraine-prone person is put in a stressful situation that frustrates his attempt to attain perfection, then blood flow to the brain can be affected. This, in turn, leads to a migraine headache.

Researchers have found that those with the emotional predisposition toward migraines can contract these very painful headaches as a result of prolonged exposure to stressors and emotional upheaval. In addition, certain foods, including chicken liver, yogurt, and some cheeses may precipitate migraine attacks. Two common triggers are the fear of failure and the undertaking of a new, very difficult, and time-consuming task.

Backaches

Backaches often are caused when the back muscles continually experience spasms—sudden, violent contractions. Medical researchers have found that back spasms are one of the most common stress-related physical complaints. Studies show that most chronic muscle spasms in the back are not brought about by overstraining through heavy lifting or other physical exertion, but by a series of physiological responses to psychological problems.

Some people keep their back muscles in a semi-contracted, tense position for months—and sometimes even years—at a time, even when they are sleeping. If the back muscles stay in this contracted position for too long, they lose their flexibility and become ineffective and weak. This brings pain when the muscle is called upon to perform even minor tasks such as bending over.

Premenstrual Pain

Many women experience a range of physical ills just prior to menstruation. There is a complex relationship between the secretion of hormones and the amount of stress a woman is under prior to menstruation. It appears as if stress is at least a part of the reason for premenstrual problems, which include nausea, swelling of the extremities, inflammation of the breasts, and headaches. Not all women suffer from these problems, and some suffer from them only periodically. But doctors have discovered that many women can avoid most of this premenstrual pain if they control their stress intake. This also is true with respect to two other female reproductive problems: lack of menstrual flow and menstrual irregularities.

Ulcerative Colitis

This disease of the colon, in which the bodily fluids eat through the colon's walls and the colon begins to bleed, results in uncontrollable and bloody bowel movements. Doctors have made the assumption that this form of colitis may be an example of the body turning on itself caused at least in part by a person who keeps hostility and anger bottled up. Those who suffer from diarrhea or constipation are experiencing less severe but similar colon problems. And there is medical evidence that anxiety, nervousness, and tension also contribute to these dysfunctions of the bowels.

Allergies

Asthma, hay fever, and even colds are all allergic diseases. During times of major stress, about 15 percent of the population is likely to come down with some type of allergic ailment. Some allergies lay dormant for years, but a sustained stressful experience can bring them on. Psychologists think that most allergic reactions actually are the physical emergence of deep-seated emotional problems that occurred in childhood.

Insomnia

In nearly all cases, the inability to sleep, insomnia, is caused by psychological stress. There are two basic types of insomnia, sleep-onset and early-awakening. In sleep-onset insomnia, the person simply cannot fall asleep. The harder he tries to fall asleep, the more difficult it is to achieve sleep. Usually, after 20 minutes or so of struggling, the sufferer gives up and resorts to a sleeping pill or any number of other activities, such as reading, eating, or watching television.

There are two basic types of sleep-onset insomnia—muscular and emotional. When you lie in bed and your body is relaxed, but your thoughts are racing, you have emotional sleep-onset insomnia. If it's the other way around—if your body is rigid, restless, and tense, but your mind is calm—then you're suffering from muscular sleep-onset insomnia.

If you have muscular insomnia, you can count sheep all night and your muscles won't relax. There is simply too much tension stored in them—tension more than likely caused by your body's inability to deal with stressors. If you have emotional insomnia, then counting sheep or some other mind-relaxing technique probably will eventually induce sleep.

Early-awakening insomnia is usually associated with depression. Usually the sufferer will get up between 3:30

and 4:30 in the morning and not be able to fall back to sleep.

Cancer

Cancer researchers are the first to admit that they cannot explain the exact causes of the many and varied types of cancer. It is known that certain agents, including radiation, toxic chemicals, viruses, and severe injuries can cause cancer. But there is also medical evidence that some persons may have what psychologists call a cancer-prone personality.

Clinical psychologist Lawrence LeShan of the Institute of Applied Biology in New York, is the leading researcher in this field. LeShan has found a set of psychological traits in cancer patients that are not found in a comparable group of noncancer patients. A large percentage of cancer patients just prior to their diagnosis experienced some type of lost relationship. Many of the cancer patients were unable to express hostility; many felt unworthy and self-hate, and experienced tensions over the relationship with one or both parents.

This chapter has sketched the relationship between stress and a variety of physical ailments. Now we will look at how stressors also can contribute to psychological problems.

4 / Emotional, Psychological, and Social Consequences of Stress

The inability to cope with a stressful life-style can contribute to many psychological, emotional, and habit-control problems. The three most prevalent stress-induced psychological and emotional problems are anxiety, anger, and depression. The most common habit-control problems include alcoholism, drug abuse, obesity, and cigarette and caffeine addiction. Those who develop emotional or habit-control problems as a result of being unable to cope effectively with the stressors of life risk having their lives dominated by the problem.

Anxiety

One of the most common emotional problems associated with stress is anxiety—a state of mental tension in which a person feels ill at ease for no specific reason. The anxiety-ridden person also is constantly worrying that something terrible is about to happen. All of us at times have our anxious moments. But the chronically anxious person experiences these feelings most of the time.

Many anxious persons also suffer from a host of psychosomatic conditions, including sweaty palms, difficulty in breathing, heart palpitations, a tingling sensation in the skin, frequent need to urinate, and muscle tension. Anxious persons, moreover, are often very moody and irritable. They typically will fly into an angry rage for seemingly trivial reasons or overreact to something pleasurable. Mood swings like this also typically result in insomnia—usually of the early-awakening variety.

There are two basic causes of anxiety in adults. Both have to do with how anxious persons perceive the world around them. The first cause is the perception—either conscious or subconscious—of life's inconsistencies. This can come about, for example, when the person—who considers herself a kind, selfless individual—uncharacteristically goes "out of character," and acts unkindly toward a friend or relative. The second basic source of anxiety of adults is the individual's constant feeling of uncertainty about life. The anxious person often does not know for sure what to expect next from life.

How does anxiety affect behavior? Most anxiety-ridden persons act in one of two extreme ways. They either retreat into a shell and become afraid to try anything new, or—on the opposite extreme—they disregard rationality during stressful situations, and take foolhardy chances. They thereby invite failure, which usually comes their way eventually. Either way, the anxiety-ridden person lives a painful life.

Anger

Another emotion closely associated with the stressors of daily life is anger. Anger results from the frustrations and

31

conflicts each of us faces every day. Anger is an emotion, like anxiety, which is a direct offshoot of how we perceive the world. Remember the fight-or-flight syndrome? Anger is our modern-day "fight" reaction to a stressful event. But it is very rare, indeed, that an angry outburst is followed by the physical release of an actual fight. The anger that we feel in a stressful situation is therefore either turned inward, or directed outward in oral abuse—usually at someone close to us and usually to the detriment of a valued relationship.

There are several physiological signs attached to anger. These include a lessening of the heart rate, an increase in blood pressure, and a tightening of muscle tension, especially in the jaw. As we have seen, these physical changes can contribute to a wide variety of painful and dangerous physical ailments. The longer we remain angry, the more likely it is that we will come down with a stress-related illness.

Depression

Psychologists suggest that depression is the emotional problem most closely related to stress. Anyone who has experienced a bout of depression does not need to be reminded that it is a mood in which you feel gloomy and dejected, and for the sufferer, the world holds nothing but hopelessness and futility.

Depression should not be confused with *disappointment*. All of us have occasions when we felt disappointed about something in our lives—not getting an expected promotion at work, or getting a flat tire on a busy highway during a snowstorm. Disappointment, unlike depression, is a feeling that is related directly to an everyday situation. Depression, on the other hand, is a much more all-encompassing state, and usually is not brought about by a single event. We all snap out of our disappointments, sometimes within minutes. Sometimes, it can take years to recover from a bout of depression.

Depression affects people differently, ranging in form from mild to severe. Most people, while depressed, cannot summon the energy to take part in any activity nor concentrate on difficult mental tasks.

Psychoanalysts think depression is caused by turning the feelings of anger inward. This theory holds that the depressed person blames himself for all of the world's problems, and then just gives up. Other psychological theories hold that depression results when a person is unable to live up to a self-imposed strict standard of personal behavior.

There are other, nonstress-related, causes of depression. These include grief over the death or rejection of a loved one. But the fact remains that in most cases, a person lapses into a depressive state immediately following a succession of stressful experiences in life such as a change of marital status, a sexual problem, a serious illness, or even moving from one city to another.

Alcoholism

Drinking alcohol in moderate amounts can help some people cope with the stressors of life. In small doses—a glass of wine or a bottle of beer in the evening, for example—alcohol relaxes inhibitions, lightens the load of stress, and often makes people gregarious. Some doctors even "prescribe" to some overworked patients a glass of beer or wine at the end of a particularly hard day.

But there is a crucial difference between occasionally drinking moderate amounts of alcohol and the compulsive heavy drinking known as alcoholism. In large amounts, alcohol becomes a deadly drug. It is a chemical depressant that destroys brain cells, attacks the heart muscles, and interferes with the body's natural immune system. Alcohol also suppresses, controls, and inhibits actions, thoughts, and feelings. Large amounts of alcohol consumed over long periods of time wear down all the body's organs. Many alcoholics wind up with serious cases of liver, brain, or nervous system damage.

Those who become alcoholics usually are initially attracted to drinking because it gives them a shot of courage and self-confidence to face the stressors of everyday life. But this is merely self-delusion. The fact is that alcohol actually inhibits your ability to handle stress. Heavy drinking is a crutch that prevents you from coping with reality. One reason why alcoholics become dependent on alcohol is that they discover that they cannot cope with life *without* the numbing effects of drinking.

Drug Abuse

The motivations that cause a person to turn to alcohol are the same as those used by those who turn to other drugs commonly abused in our society: antidepressants, sedatives, stimulants, hallucinogens, marijuana, and narcotics.

Americans have been using drugs to relieve themselves of psychic and physical pain for centuries. Patent medicines and other concoctions of the late nineteenth century contained various combinations of alcohol, cocaine, heroin, and morphine. We owe the present stage of drug abuse largely to developments that began in the mid-1950s when a series of new drugs was developed to help make life easier for patients in mental hospitals. Since then, milder forms of these drugs have been developed to treat those with much less severe psychiatric troubles.

The most popular way to reduce stress is to take a drug. Drugs have become for millions of Americans the easy answer to the problems of stress. A sleeping pill at night to ward off insomnia. A pep pill the next morning to get going again. An antidepressant to cure the blues.

The continual, regular use of drugs, either willingly, or unwillingly due to physical or psychological addiction, is certainly *not* the answer to the problems associated with stress. This form of drug abuse creates more problems for the user than it solves.

The most commonly abused drugs today are prescription tranquilizers and sedatives. The two most popular tranquilizers—the antianxiety drugs called Valium and Librium, are used by millions to put off feelings of anxiety. Others form an attachment to barbiturates such as Seconal.

Another class of abused drugs is the stimulants, including amphetamines and cocaine. Doctors have prescribed an amphetamine, Ritalin, to treat hyperactive children. But adults are the prime abusers of stimulants such as Dexedrine and Benzedrine—so-called pep pills, which give people a lift and extra energy. These drugs, if taken continuously, can cause physical addiction. They also give the user a tolerance, meaning that larger and larger doses are needed to achieve the desired effect. Some abusers of stimulants wind up injecting the drugs into their blood-streams, a type of destructive behavior that can result in a severe mental disease called amphetamine psychosis.

LSD and other hallucinogenic drugs such as mescaline and peyote, which unlike the amphetamines and barbiturates cannot be obtained legally, had a measure of popularity in the late 1960s and early 1970s. Small segments of the population continue to use them today. A continuing problem, though, especially among young persons, is marijuana abuse. Although marijuana has no known major physiological side effects, constant use of the drug can lead to the same physical problems associated with tobacco use—especially lung and heart problems.

While healthy adults usually are able to smoke moderate

amounts of marijuana without endangering their health, there is plenty to worry about with the narcotic drugs, such as morphine and heroin. Most of us don't need to be reminded that these drugs are powerfully addictive. Users who try to kick heroin, morphine, or other narcotic habits are forced to go through painful and dangerous periods of physical withdrawal.

Cocaine, the chemically treated active ingredient of the coca leaf, is classified by the government as a narcotic. But in pharmacological terms, cocaine is a stimulant that acts on the central nervous system, speeding up the heart and the brain. There has been a rapid increase in the number of people using cocaine in this country in recent years. This new "social drug," its users claim, helps them cope with stressful situations and just makes life more enjoyable.

But with the increase of cocaine use has come a parallel increase in cocaine abuse. Admissions to emergency rooms for cocaine problems have risen dramatically in the last five years. And some well-known persons—including those in the entertainment and sports fields—have fallen victim to the drug's addictive properties. Cocaine, in the strict sense of the word, is not physically addictive. But using large amounts of the pure drug (usually by treating it with chemicals to get to its base and then smoking the free base) creates a psychological craving for the drug that is nearly impossible to overcome.

Caffeine

The most widely used stimulant in this country is not illegal. In fact, anyone can purchase large quantities of it at any grocery store. The stimulant in question is caffeine, which is found in coffee, tea, chocolate, cola drinks, and other soft drinks, and is added to some prescription and nonprescription drugs.

Like the other stimulants, caffeine acts on the central nervous system and increases the heart rate, while functioning as a diuretic. Used in moderate amounts, caffeine can be beneficial to those faced with boring or monotonous jobs, since the drug helps to keep you alert, think clearly, and concentrate on the tasks at hand.

But like other drugs, caffeine brings with it the potential for abuse. Many persons cannot function without two or three cups of coffee in the morning, a few more cups in the afternoon, and a cola drink or two thrown in during the day. Doctors have found that such excessive caffeine consumption may be linked to a host of harmful ailments including heart disease, birth defects, digestive disorders, a benign breast disorder called fibrocystic disease, and even cancer.

Caffeine, too, can contribute to anxiety. Someone who consumes large amounts of caffeine every day will feel anxious when he tries to cut back on caffeine consumption. These anxious feelings often are accompanied by physical withdrawal symptoms, including severe headaches, nausea, and vomiting. It's clear that those with problems coping with stressors should avoid consuming large amounts of caffeine.

Obesity

For nearly all Americans, eating has very little to do with hunger. Americans tend to overeat every day, and not surprisingly, many of us are overweight. If you have any doubt about that statement, take a look at the list of today's best-selling books. It's a good bet you'll find a few offering advice on diet and weight loss.

There is a difference between being overweight and being obese. Obesity—exceeding your desirable weight by at least twenty percent—is a potentially dangerous condition that doctors believe leads to a range of illnesses, most notably heart disease. Being overweight also is unhealthy, but is not as precipitously dangerous to your health as is being obese.

There are a number of different charts that list desirable weight by age, sex, height, and bone structure. But there is a much easier way to see if you are obese or overweight. Just take a look at your naked body in the mirror. You'll know immediately if you are obese. If you see excessive amounts of bodily fat on your upper arms, thighs, and across your abdominal area, you are obese. If, when you grab your skin around your midsection or your upper arm between your thumb and forefinger and come up with at least an inch of fat, you're overweight.

The main reason why most of us are overweight is very simple. We eat too much. And nearly all of us overeat as a way of coping with stressors. Just as the Type A person reacts to pressure by overworking, and the alcoholic reacts to stressors and pressure by turning to the bottle, obese and overweight persons turn to food as a crutch against the stress of everyday life.

There are a few other stress-related problems involving oral habits. One is anorexia nervosa, a condition that usually is found among teenage girls who choose to starve themselves rather than overeat. Closely related is a condition known as bulimia, in which the person—again, usually a young woman—goes on binges of eating large amounts of food and then vomiting immediately afterward.

Cigarette Smoking

Cigarette smoking is another unhealthy practice that people choose to take part in for reasons that have to do with stress. There are other reasons why people smoke— peer pressure among young persons, for example. And some say that they smoke simply because they enjoy the taste of cigarettes.

But tens of millions of people smoke as a way to cope with stressors. Smokers use the acts of lighting up, inhaling, and exhaling to relax during times of stress, and as a way of combating nervousness. Even most cigarette smokers are aware of the known health consequences of cigarette smoking: an increasing risk of developing lung cancer, emphysema, and heart disease.

Social Consequences of the Stressful Life-style

These varied emotional problems—from anxiety to obesity—associated with stress can contribute to a host of social consequences. We've already discussed a few of the social consequences, such as the problems involved when a person cannot control his anger and lashes out at friends or relatives. The other social consequences stemming from emotional problems are similar. They often can put severe strains on marital relationships and social relationships and make life miserable for co-workers.

Social action itself can even contribute to stress-related mental and physical problems. The opportunities for stress are most present in family and marriage situations. These interpersonal relationships should in the best of all possible worlds be the places where we can relax and not face any of the stress-producing events of life. But many persons' personal lives actually *produce* the stressors that lead to the physical and emotional problems we've been describing.

Let's look at marriage. Spousal relationships bring with them the comfort and security of love and acceptance— but they also bring inevitable moments of conflict that can cause stress. The death or severe illness of a spouse, divorce, or separation—these are all problem areas that can be stressful. It is also not uncommon to see long-term married couples involved in constant, unresolved conflicts that also act as stressors.

Among the other stressful situations inherent in family life are child rearing, money problems, moving, and lack of communication. These are the most common family problem areas. Without all members of the family dealing with these problems openly, they can lead to the emotional and physical stress-induced problems we've described.

Those who live alone, whether they are unmarried, separated, divorced, or widowed, also face a set of potentially stressful problem areas. Psychologists say that the most important coping mechanism for those living alone is to have a network of friends and relatives who can be depended upon for help in potentially stressful situations—anything from being alone on a Saturday night to helping arrange the details of a parent's funeral.

Stress on the Job

It is only natural that the stresses of life manifest themselves on the job. Psychologists claim that most of the emotional problems of employees do not originate in the workplace, but these problems affect job performance because they typically lead to declining work performance, including excessive lateness, absenteeism, on-the-job accidents, and failure to get along with co-workers.

This is not to say that our jobs themselves do not present us with potentially stressful opportunities. They do. It's not difficult to see what causes stress at work: innate conflicts between workers and supervisors, conflicts with co-workers, unhappiness with one's job, fear of being replaced, and worries about advancing up the career ladder.

Emotional, Psychological, and Social Consequences

The common stereotype of the overworked, unhealthy, pressured executive being the person who is subjected to the greatest amount of stress is not exactly correct. Yes, some high-powered, high-pressure executives work too hard, smoke too much, are overweight, don't watch their diets, and refuse to exercise. But it turns out that many of those who rise to high positions in the corporate world also have the ability to fight off the stressors of life. They are survivors; they manage to control their lives and wind up handling their stress-related problems adequately.

Secretaries, assembly-line workers, middle managers, and clerical workers—those who are trying to work their way to the top or those who are struggling with menial jobs—these are the workers who are subjected to the highest levels of job-induced stress. These are the people who are under the most time constraints and tend to be the most overworked. And, as should be obvious, these are the persons who are most prone to stress-induced psychosomatic illnesses.

Some workers experience a stress-related syndrome called job burnout. This occurs, for example, when a social worker with 250 cases is assigned 50 additional cases because of budget and staff cutbacks. The social worker becomes frustrated by the volume of the work he must handle every day, and one day, just gives up.

Burnout is a stress response to overwork, poor supervision, and unpleasant working surroundings. The worker with job burnout often exhibits many of the emotional and physical reactions associated with stress.

Every time we start a new job, we put ourselves under extremely stress-provoking situations. This problem is compounded when the new job is in a new part of the country. Any type of relocation is fraught with stressors. The stressors involved in physical relocation include today's uncertain housing market with high mortgage rates and exorbitant rents, and the uprooting of children from friends and schoolmates. Some employees consider relocation tantamount to a demotion, and work to avoid a move, especially if it involves going to a part of the country where the cost of living is much higher than where they are.

5 / Self-Trait Inventory

This chapter will help you test your own level of stress by using two inventories to better understand some of the warning signs. The inventories catalog your personality traits and measure how they cause stress.

Let's talk a bit about personality before going over the individual personality traits. Volumes have been written on the human *personality,* yet the psychiatric community does not even agree on a simple definition of the word. The ancient Greeks studied personality and came up with four types: the *sanguine* person who is happy and optimistic; the *choleric* person who is bad-tempered; the *melancholy* person who is moody; and the *phlegmatic* person who is listless.

Each of these conditions the Greeks believed was caused by a person's bodily fluids. Richly flowing red blood was supposed to cause the sanguine person's happiness. An excess of yellow bile supposedly caused the choleric personality, an excess of black bile the melancholy, and an excess of phlegm, the phlegmatic.

No one believes in the bile and blood theory of personality today. But psychologists do believe that biological factors—including brain structure, hormone production, and body type—do influence our personalities. And, so too, do

43

social factors. But whatever causes the makeup of the personality—which we can broadly define as the consistent pattern of behavior including thinking and feeling that a person exhibits when confronting different situations—are not constant. We can and do exhibit a wide range of thoughts, feelings, and responses depending on the situations we face in life.

Which brings us to how our personality traits can determine the extent and cause of stress. Most psychologists now believe that what happens to us—the external conditions that we face every day—has at least the same effect on our personality makeup as do those factors present in our internal psychological makeup.

A good way to find out exactly which external factors (stressors) are influencing your personality traits is to keep a special weekly diary. In this diary, you divide each day into three periods—morning, afternoon, and evening. Within those periods there's space for you to set down the major events that take place—whether they are highlights or lowlights, or anything in between. Alongside those events you describe the personality trait you exhibited. We provide a long list of personality traits so you can catalog each one as positive or negative.

If you keep the diary for seven days, you should see a pattern emerge. You'll see exactly where clusters of positive and negative personality traits come from. This will give you a basis for figuring out a strategy to try to lessen your stress load.

What follows is a list of personality traits, arranged alphabetically. They cover a wide range of emotions, but of course cannot describe exactly every emotion you will feel during the week. So, if what you're feeling is not on the list, write it down anyway, and later compare it to the listed traits. You should be able to tell quite readily whether the trait is positive or negative.

After the list of personality traits is a daily diary filled out recently by a twenty-eight-year-old working mother during a typical Friday. Use this as a guide for your own daily diaries. We provide blank diaries for you, or you can draw up your own if there is not enough space on the ones provided.

Positive Personality Traits

Absorbed	Cool	Flexible	Merry
Adamant	Cooperative	Friendly	Mirthful
Adventurous	Curious	Fulfilled	Moved
Affectionate	Daring	Glad	Mystical
Alert	Dazzled	Good-Humored	Nice
Alive	Delighted	Grateful	Nutty
Amazed	Desirous	Gratified	Optimistic
Amused	Determined	Happy	Open
Animated	Dominant	Heavenly	Overjoyed
Appreciative	Eager	Helpful	Peaceful
Aroused	Ecstatic	Hopeful	Pleasant
Assertive	Effervescent	High	Pleased
Astonished	Elated	Honored	Pretty
Awed	Electrified	Immortal	Proud
Beautiful	Enchanted	Impressed	Quiet
Blissful			
Bold	Encouraged	Infatuated	Radiant
Brave	Energetic	Inquisitive	Rapturous
Buoyant	Enervated	Inspired	Refreshed
Calm	Engrossed	Intense	Relaxed
Capable	Enjoyment	Interested	Relieved
Carefree	Enlivened	Intrigued	Reverent
Charmed	Enthusiastic	Invigorated	Rewarded
Cheated	Exalted	Involved	Righteous
Cheerful	Excited	Joyful	Sated
Clever	Exhilarated	Jubilant	Satisfied
Comfortable	Expansive	Keyed Up	Secure
Complacent	Expectant	Kicky	Sensitive
Composed	Exuberant	Kind	Sexy
Concerned	Fascinated	Loving	Spellbound
Confident	Free	Mellow	Splendid

ALIVE & WELL STRESS BOOK
Positive Personality Traits

Stimulated	Tender	Trusting	Wonderful
Sure	Thankful	Vital	Zany
Surprised	Thrilled	Vivacious	
Sympathetic	Touched	Warm	
Talkative	Tranquil	Wide-Awake	

Negative Personality Traits

Abandoned	Competitive	Displeased	Grief
Afraid	Concerned	Disquieted	Guilty
Aggravated	Condemned	Dissatisfied	Gullible
Agitated	Confused	Distracted	Hate
Agonized	Conspicuous	Distraught	Heavy
Alarmed	Contrite	Distressed	Helpless
Aloof	Cool	Disturbed	Hesitant
Ambivalent	Credulous	Divided	Homesick
Angry	Critical	Dominated	Hopeless
Anguished	Cross	Downcast	Horrible
Animosity	Cruel	Dubious	Horrified
Annoyance	Crushed	Embittered	Hostile
Anxiety	Culpable	Empty	Hot
Apathetic	Deceitful	Envious	Humdrum
Apprehensive	Dejected	Evil	Hurt
Argumentative	Depressed	Exasperated	Hysterical
Aroused	Despondent	Exhausted	Ignored
Beat	Destructive	Fatigued	Impatient
Betrayed	Detached	Fauning	Imposed Upon
Bitter	Different	Fearful	Indifferent
Blah	Diffident	Fidgety	Inefficient
Blue	Diminished	Flustered	Inert
Bored	Disappointed	Foolish	Infuriated
Breathless	Discouraged	Forlorn	Inquisitive
Brokenhearted	Disgruntled	Frantic	Insecure
Burdened	Disgusted	Frightened	Insensitive
Captivated	Disheartened	Frustrated	Intense
Chagrined	Disinterested	Furious	Intimidated
Challenged	Dislike	Gloomy	Introverted
Cold	Dismayed	Greedy	Isolated

Self-Trait Inventory
Negative Personality Traits

Irate	Nutty	Sad	Tempted
Irked	Obnoxious	Scared	Tenacious
Irritated	Obsessed	Screwed Up	Tense
Jealous	Odd	Sensitive	Tenuous
Jittery	Opposed	Shaky	Terrified
Jumpy	Outraged	Shocked	Terrible
Laconic	Pained	Silly	Threatened
Lazy	Panicked	Skeptical	Thwarted
Lecherous	Persecuted	Sleepy	Timid
Letdown	Pessimistic	Sneaky	Tired
Lethargic	Possessive	Solemn	Troubled
Licentious	Provoked	Sorrowful	Trapped
Listless	Petrified	Sorry	Ugly
Lonely	Pity	Sour	Uncooperative
Longing	Precarious	Spiritless	Uneasy
Low	Pressured	Spiteful	Unfriendly
Lustful	Prim	Startled	Unhappy
Mad	Prissy	Stingy	Unnerved
Maudlin	Puzzled	Stuffed	Unsteady
Mean	Quarrelsome	Stunned	Uptight
Melancholy	Reluctant	Stupefied	Vexed
Miserable	Remorseful	Submissive	Violent
Mopey	Repelled	Suffering	Vulnerable
Naughty	Resentful	Surprised	Worried
Nervous	Restless	Suspicious	

DIARY OF PERSONALITY TRAITS

	Event	Personality Trait Exhibited	Positive	Negative
Day 1	Wake up early: 5:30 A.M.	Fretful		✓
Morning	Daughter and I prepare for day	Excited	✓	
	Took bus/subway to work	Dull, tiring		✓
	Walked from subway to office	Pleasant (creative thoughts)	✓	
	Worked on schedule	Calm	✓	
Afternoon	Lunch with new staffer	Interested	✓	
	Walked back to office	Unsettled (want day to end).		✓
	In office (easy afternoon workload)	Claustrophobic		✓
		Happy, silly	✓	
	Office party	Happy, energetic	✓	
Evening	Missed scheduled tennis game	Disappointed		✓
	Dinner with friend	Contented	✓	
	Movie	Bored, sleepy		✓

SECTION

II

Stress Reducers

The first section covered stress producers. Now we will take a look at stress reducers—ways to alleviate stress. This includes physical relaxation techniques, meditation, yoga, exercise, deep breathing, and proper diet and nutrition.

We are taking a holistic approach to stress reduction—an approach that involves treating the whole person, the mind and the body, without resorting to drugs.

Any one of the techniques we present will help you ward off the detrimental effects of stress. Read through each one, and then choose one or more routines that you think suit your personal life-style. Or, you can pick and choose parts of each of the stress reducers and work them into a special antistress routine of your own.

6 / Learning How to Relax

There are a host of proven relaxation techniques, all of which fight the effects of stress. This is because the body's response to relaxation is the opposite of its response to stress. Relaxation induces a number of physical changes that counteract stress. These include a lowering of the heartbeat, a lessening of muscle tension, and lowered levels of blood pressure and cholesterol in the blood. Best of all, those who practice relaxation techniques report a lessening of mental tension and a pleasant general feeling in mind and body.

There are two basic types of relaxation techniques—physical and emotional. The next few chapters provide detailed instructions on how you can practice techniques of both types. Some find relief from stress by combining the two types into a personalized program. Feel free to integrate parts of any of the following relaxation routines into your own personal program. Just be sure to give yourself time—at least two weeks of daily practice—before discarding one technique in favor of another.

Learning how to relax is a skill. And as is the case with other skills, it takes discipline and regular practice to master it properly. We therefore recommend that those embarking on the relaxation program outlined in this chapter, try to do two 30-minute sessions every day for a month. This won't be easy, especially at first. But if you stick with the routine, you should soon begin to see results. If you continue to do the relaxation exercises regularly, you should notice a significant difference in all aspects of your life after about 10 weeks of practice. You will feel and look relaxed. Your arms and legs will hang loosely; your facial muscles also will relax; your skin will be smoother and less wrinkled. And, best of all, you will have a new relaxed, calm outlook that will help you combat the effects of a stressful life-style.

After you've achieved these results, you may want to cut back your relaxation regimen to a single daily 30-minute session. But if you find that one session does not do the trick, or if you get pleasure from your two daily sessions, by all means keep up the two-a-day routine.

A Relaxation Routine
(A Half-Hour Program)

It's important for you to wear comfortable clothing when you do relaxation exercises. If you plan to do the routine during your working day, simply take off your shoes and loosen the clothes around your stomach, neck, and chest. If you have a chance to change, it's best to wear a loose-fitting T-shirt and gym shorts or a sweat suit or warm-up suit or a leotard.

Find a quiet spot to do your relaxation routine. Dim the lights. You may want to play some quiet classical music. But most people prefer absolute quiet.

Before starting the relaxation exercises, take a few minutes to do some standing stretches. This will make it easier for you to begin to relax your muscles once you start the routine. Stand with your feet shoulder-length apart, and reach both hands up toward the ceiling. Stretch out until you feel a slight strain. Then release the tension, and let your arms drop slowly toward the floor. Hold that position for a few seconds, and then stretch up again. Drop your arms down once again, and repeat the routine a third time.

While you're standing, try a few more loosening-up exercises. Extend your arms away from your body at shoulder level. Stand still and swing your extended left arm back to the left while at the same time swinging your extended right arm across your body in front of you in the same direction. Stop when you feel the slightest tension. Then swing both arms in the opposite direction. Keep swinging your arms back and forth for about 20–30 seconds. Then release any residual tension in your arms and wrists by shaking your hands vigorously. As you do this, pretend there's something sticking to your hands and you're trying to shake it off.

Now take a minute or two to loosen up your shoulders. Stand still and make exaggerated shrugs of your shoulders, pointing your shoulders up toward your ears. Hold the shrug for a few seconds, and then let your shoulders drop. Next, reach down with your hands toward the floor, and let your shoulders drop in the opposite direction. Alternate the shrugging and the dropping for about 30 seconds.

Next try some neck stretching. For this, sit down and get comfortable. Close your eyes. Sit up straight. Drop your chin toward your chest, letting your head fall forward comfortably. Do not overstrain. It's a good idea to exhale as you do so. Then, inhale and raise your head, and let it fall back as far as you can comfortably. Hold it there a second or two, and repeat the forward-backward movement 5 more times.

Now bring your head back to the center and try to touch your left ear to your left shoulder. Do not raise or lower your shoulders, and do not overstrain. When you feel the slightest tension in your neck, stop. Now, bring your head back to the center, and try to touch your right ear to your right shoulder. Repeat the ear-to-shoulder movements 5 more times.

Now open your eyes and turn your head all the way to the right and try to see directly behind you. Don't move any other part of your body. Hold your head there for a second, bring it back to center, and then look over your left shoulder behind your back. Hold it there for another second and return to the center. Try this 5 more times.

Now you're ready for full neck rolls. Close your eyes again, and drop your chin to your chest, inhale, and roll your right ear over to your right shoulder. Remember not to move anything but the head and neck. Pay careful attention to your shoulders. Don't allow them to sag or rise. Now exhale and swing your head back, then inhale and roll it over, bringing the left ear to the left shoulder. Keep your eyes closed during the full neck rolls. Keep breathing deeply, concentrating on your neck muscles and your breathing. When you've completed a few rolls in the clockwise direction, roll your neck a few more times counterclockwise.

If you feel any dizziness at any time, stop. Take a few deep breaths. Don't do any more neck rolls until the dizziness is gone.

After these few stretching exercises you are ready for the relaxation routine based on tensing and relaxing the muscles. The routine may be done either lying on your back on a bed or on a well-padded rug, or sitting in a chair. The main thing is to make sure you are comfortable. You want to be very comfortable, but you don't want to go to sleep. Remember, you are working at learning a new and somewhat difficult skill, the art of relaxation. While you do the exercises, try to put all thoughts about everything else—your job, your spouse, your children, your friends, and family—out of your head. Concentrate only on the exercise you are doing at the moment.

Chapter 11 contains a comprehensive lesson in deep-breathing techniques, complete with a number of specific deep-breathing exercises. The breathing you have to do during relaxation exercises you can learn in 5 minutes. This type of breathing, called abdominal or diaphragmatic breathing, serves as a giant helping hand as you try to relax the muscles.

During the day, most of us breathe shallowly, using only the nose, throat, and chest. A deep, diaphragmatic breath, on the other hand, begins in the abdomen. In this manner, the maximal amount of stale air is pushed out of the body as you exhale, and the maximal amount of fresh air is brought in when you inhale.

Try taking a diaphragmatic breath. Keep your mouth closed, and breathe through the nostrils. Put your right hand on your stomach and inhale deeply. If you are breathing diaphragmatically, your stomach should expand like a balloon as you inhale, and then contract as you exhale. If your stomach isn't moving, you're breathing too shallowly. Push lightly with your hand into your stomach as you exhale to train yourself to breathe from the abdomen. It is essential to learn this method of deep breathing in order to get the full benefit not only from the relaxation exercises, but also from meditation and yoga.

Now that you've learned the basics of abdominal breathing, you can begin the relaxation routine. You should be sitting or lying down. Close your eyes. Feel your surroundings. Center yourself. Now take 2 deep, slow diaphragmatic breaths. Inhale slowly to the count of 3, repeating to yourself "1, 1,000, 2, 1,000, 3, 1,000." Hold that breath for 3 more seconds, and then slowly exhale to the count of 3. As you exhale, try to visualize all the tensions of your body leaving along with the stale air. As you inhale, concentrate on the invigorating, clean fresh air you are bringing into your body.

After taking 2 deep breaths, relax for a few seconds, letting your breathing return to normal. Then take a large inhalation, and as you do so, simultaneously stretch and tense up all the muscles in the body as hard as you can. This won't be easy to do at first. It's an awkward and unfamiliar movement. But try it nonetheless. After a week or so of practicing, you'll get the hang of it.

Hold the full body inhalation and stretch for just about 2 seconds. Feel the tension. Then begin a long exhalation and gently allow all your muscles to relax. Again, as you exhale, try to visualize the stale air and tension you are expelling from your body.

Keep your eyes closed during the whole routine, and think about only what you are doing. Next, you will begin to alternately tense and then relax all of your major muscle groups. As you do so, you will be inhaling as you tense up, and exhaling as you relax. To repeat: As you inhale, your stomach expands like a balloon; as you exhale, your stomach muscles draw in. Try not to let your mind wander during the relaxation exercises; concentrate only on the muscles you are working on.

Start with your right hand and arm. Clench your right first, squeezing it tightly. As you hold the tension, concentrate on your entire right arm. Hold your fist tensed for 5 seconds, and then slowly release it. As you release, exhale and picture all the tension in your right arm leaving your body along with the exhalation. Compare the feeling in your fingers, fist, wrist, and arm when tensed, and when relaxed. Now repeat the whole process. Make a tense fist, hold it tight for 5 seconds, and then relax and let your entire right arm go limp. Do this routine twice with your left arm.

Now tense up your shoulders by using the same shrugging motion you used while warming up. Hold your shoulders tensed up toward your ears for 5 seconds, then slowly exhale, release, and relax. Repeat a second time.

Next push your neck back into the floor, mattress, or chair to tense it up. Be careful not to overstrain, but don't baby yourself either. Feel the tension in your neck as you hold it for 5 seconds. Then exhale and relax your neck totally. If you're sitting in a chair, let your neck hang limply forward for a second or two. If you're lying down, release all the pressure in your neck and rest.

It's a good idea to repeat the neck exercise 2 or 3 more times because a lot of us hold a great deal of tension in our neck muscles. Take extra time with the exercise if you feel you need it. When you're finished, do a few easy neck rolls to release the remaining tension. Now just relax for a few seconds, and feel what you've done to your arms, shoulders, and neck. They should be thoroughly and completely relaxed.

Now it's time to work on the jaw muscles. Clench your teeth for 5 seconds, and then relax. Try not to tighten the neck muscles or any other muscles of the body when you are clenching your jaw. Remember to concentrate solely on the jaw. Repeat the jaw clench a second time, hold it for 5 seconds, and then relax.

Now open your mouth as wide as you can without overstraining. Hold it there for 5 seconds, and then relax it totally. Open your mouth very wide again. This time stick out your tongue as far as you can. Hold it out there for 5 seconds, and then close your mouth and relax your tongue. One more time: Open your mouth, stick out your tongue (remember to try to keep all your other facial muscles relaxed), and this time point your tongue toward your head and then toward your toes before you relax totally.

Now work on your eyes. Remember again to keep all your other facial muscles relaxed. If you tense them, you won't be getting enough relaxation into the eye muscles.

Open your eyes as wide as you can. Hold them open for 5 seconds. Then close them and squint tightly. Hold that squint shut tightly for 5 more seconds, then relax. Repeat the eye tensing and relaxing once more, concentrating only on the eyes. Don't move your lips or clench your jaw.

The next facial muscles are in the forehead. To tense the muscles in your brow, pretend you're very unhappy, and force your face into an exaggerated frown. When you do this, you should feel your forehead tense up. Hold the tension for the requisite 5 seconds, then relax. Now tense up your brow a little differently, by raising your eyebrows as high as they'll go and feel the tension. Lower your eyebrows after 5 seconds and then tense them and relax again. Now all the muscles in your face and head should be completely relaxed.

At this point, you should take a short break. Without moving any part of your body, take 3 more long, exaggerated diaphragmatic breaths. Breathe in slowly to a count of 3. Hold your breath for 3 seconds, and then exhale this time to a slow count of 5. Now breathe normally without moving for at least 60 seconds.

You're now ready to work on your abdominal, back, and leg muscles. It's very easy to coordinate inhalations and exhalations while tensing and relaxing the abdominal muscles. This is because as you tense the abdominal muscles, you exaggerate an inhalation and your stomach automatically expands. So go ahead and tense up your stomach, hold it for 5 seconds, and then exhale and relax very slowly. Repeat the process one more time and breathe normally.

Next, tighten the muscles in your back by arching it stiffly. Hold the tension for 5 seconds and then exhale and relax. Repeat. Then tense all the muscles in your right leg by lifting it a few inches off the ground and stretching your big toe out as far as you can, pointing it away from you. Hold the tension in the entire leg for 5 seconds. Feel the leg get heavier and heavier. Then slowly exhale and relax the leg. Repeat once more with the right leg and twice with the left.

You've now worked on all of the major muscle groups. But you're not finished with your relaxation routine. What comes next is the most important step in the entire routine. This part is called the final relaxation in yoga, and is based on the concept of autosuggestion, a mild form of self-hypnosis. What you do is consciously tell your body parts to relax, and—miraculously—they respond to your commands.

After you finish the final leg tension-relaxation, sit still for a few minutes. Breathe normally. Then begin the autosuggestion. Keep your eyes closed. Visualize your right foot and think to yourself: "My foot is relaxed. My foot is relaxed. My foot is *completely* relaxed." Then, in sequence, visualize your right ankle, shin, and thigh, and repeat the appropriate autosuggestion to yourself as you visualize each part of the leg.

When you finish the right leg, try to visualize the entire leg and say to yourself: "My entire leg is relaxed. My entire leg is relaxed. My entire leg is *completely* relaxed." Repeat the same routine with the left leg.

Then go on to your hands and arms. Start with the fingers of the right hand, then the hand itself, the wrist, elbow, and upper arm. Then do the left hand and arm. Move on to your abdomen, your buttocks, genitals, chest, shoulders, and neck. Then, go over each part of the head—chin, jaw, eyes, and forehead.

When you've finished—and this autosuggestion routine should take about 5 minutes—say to yourself: "My entire body is relaxed. My entire body is relaxed. My entire body is *completely* relaxed."

Next comes the easiest part of the routine. You simply lie or sit motionless for 5 to 10 minutes. Keep your eyes closed. Breathe normally. Don't fall asleep. Concentrate on your breathing. You should feel totally relaxed. Your system should be slowed down to a snail's pace. Your mind should be in a pleasant, dreamlike state.

It's a good idea to use some sort of timing device to signal yourself after 10 minutes of final relaxation. If you use an alarm clock, try to find one that does not have a jarring bell or buzzer. As you come out of the final relaxation, do it slowly. Roll your head gently from side to side, keeping your eyes closed. Slowly wriggle your toes and fingers. Gently shake your legs and arms. Then sit up with your eyes still closed.

Sit still for a few seconds. Concentrate on how you feel. It's a good bet that you're now at the most relaxed point you'll be all day. Try to remember what you're feeling. With practice, you'll be able to put yourself in this state after a few minutes of relaxation any time during the day. This relaxation method is one of the few sure antidotes to life's pressures, tensions, and stress.

7 / Meditation

> The apparent effectiveness of meditation as an antidote to stress certainly makes it a desirable component in a comprehensive program for the reduction of stress.
>
> Robert L. Woolfolk and
> Frank R. Richardson,
> *Stress, Sanity & Survival.*

Numerous psychological studies in recent years have confirmed what practitioners of meditation have known for the last 2,000 years—namely, that meditation is an extremely effective method of slowing down the body and fully relaxing the mind.

Many people associate meditation with mysterious, ritualistic Eastern religions. Meditation did, in fact, begin in the East and is used by Hindus, Buddhists, and other religious groups today. But you can get all the benefits of meditation without ascribing to any religious tenets. Meditation, simply, is a discipline which when practiced brings a special state of consciousness as you concentrate your attention solely on one thought or object. Meditation for religious purposes may involve focusing on God. But meditation for relaxation purposes need not have anything to do with religion.

Historians note that Hindu monks began to use meditative techniques about 2,500 years ago. The branch of Hinduism most closely associated with meditation is yoga. The Zen Buddhists of Japan borrowed the yogic meditation concept and evolved another type of meditation, called Zen meditation. Meditation was used later on in three other Eastern religions: Shintoism (the state religion of Japan), Taoism (a Chinese offshoot of Buddhism founded by Lao-Tzu in the sixth century B.C.), and Confucianism (the teachings of the great third-century B.C. Chinese philosopher Confucius). Certain meditative practices also have been used by Jews, Christians, and Sufi Muslims.

Today, different techniques of meditation have been adopted by a host of religious groups, most of which are offshoots of traditional yoga or Zen. Most of these meditation methods have one thing in common: focusing the attention on one object—either a thought, a physical object, or a word. In some types of meditation, students are instructed to meditate with their eyes open, concentrating on an object, such as an intricately detailed geometric design with a multicolored object at its center called a mandala, or any number of other objects including statues, paintings, photographs, flowers, the sun, the stars, or a candle's flame.

Some yoga groups advocate walking meditation, usually just before dawn. During a silent group meditation walk, each person concentrates on the physical surroundings. These walks are typically held in rural areas or along a seashore. The final part of a walking meditation usually consists of a 15-minute sitting meditation in which meditators concentrate on an object in nature such as a sunrise, sunset, or waterfall. Some runners today meditate during their running workouts, repeating to themselves a word or phrase as they run.

The most common types of meditation, however, are done with the eyes closed, usually with the meditator sitting in a comfortable position. The differences in sitting, silent meditation has to do with what the meditator concentrates on. In some disciplines, the meditator concentrates on a part of his body; some Hindu sects actually do concentrate on the navel. Other branches of Hindus concentrate on what is called the third eye—a spot in the middle of the forehead that is said to contain psychic powers. Yet another group concentrates alternatively on different parts of the body. Some groups advocate concentrating on imaginary objects such as the sea, clouds, a flower, or any other calming image the mind can call up.

What exactly happens during the meditative state? Psychologists have only recently begun testing practitioners of meditation to find out. These tests have found that experienced meditators are able to bring about a series of physical changes within minutes after they begin meditating. The physiological changes are nearly identical to those that result from the physical relaxation techniques we discussed in the previous chapter. These changes can be an antidote to the harmful physical reactions to prolonged stress.

The major physiological changes induced by meditation are a decrease in the heart rate and a slowing of breath. In addition, blood pressure lowers, tension eases in the muscles, and oxygen consumption decreases due to this overall reduction in energy use as the entire body actually "slows down." It sounds like what happens to someone who is put under hypnosis. But changes differ from those that the body goes through under hypnosis because during meditation bodily processes are slowed but the meditator remains alert and awake.

Meditation, medical studies also have found, brings a temporary shutdown of the mechanisms in the brain that screen information. In addition, EEG (electroencephalogram) tests show conclusively that experienced meditators have an increase in alpha brain waves when meditating. An increased alpha brain wave flow usually occurs during sleep, and is a sign that the body is totally relaxed.

Thus far, we've painted a glowing picture of meditation. But even though nearly everyone can derive benefits from meditation, there are some who should not undertake this discipline. Some people who suffer from chronic migraine headaches have reported that meditating actually brings on a migraine. Others, including some cardiac patients, become dizzy during meditation; a few people become panic-stricken, and lose control of themselves while meditating. It should be noted that only a very few persons react negatively to meditation, but those few should not undertake a meditation program.

Nearly all of us, though, can benefit from meditation. Indeed, some migraine sufferers have reported that after learning how to meditate, they can ward off these exceedingly painful headaches.

Here's another caution before you embark on a meditation program. For many of us, sitting in one spot and trying to concentrate and rid our minds of all extraneous thoughts is the hardest thing in the world to do. Meditative concentration requires strong discipline—especially when you are just starting out. It takes patience, practice and perseverance to master what on the surface may sound like a very simple thing to do.

Psychologist Kenneth R. Pelletier described some of the problems in his book, *Mind as Healer, Mind as Slayer.*

> Mental activity is a wayward and not easily controlled phenomenon. At first, it seems to have a life of its own. When you exert will or volition and attempt to become quiet, it is very likely that you will be perversely and regularly disobeyed. Your mind jumps unbidden from one thought or

concern to another despite your efforts to concentrate on eliminating such activity. With practice and experimentation to determine the best approach for you personally, you can gradually increase your ability to regulate your attention and reduce or rectify the mind's overwhelming tendency to generate incessant activity or distraction.[1]

Pelletier and other meditation experts recommend that those who have trouble meditating consult with a trained meditation instructor. This is true especially for beginners. Some of those who cannot get comfortable in their first few meditation sessions can get frustrated, give up, and never try it again. Just remember that mental attitude is very important in this subtly difficult type of discipline. Once you cross the line and begin thinking negatively about meditation, it's exceedingly difficult to overcome those negative thoughts and start meditating successfully. And, furthermore, if you are a skeptic and do not believe that meditation will help you, the chances are that—as with other self-fulfilling prophecies—you will never succeed.

Meditation alone is not the answer to overcoming stress. But hundreds of thousands of Americans have found that meditating regularly really helps them relax and cope with the tensions in their everyday lives. By all means, attend a meditation class if you feel the need to do so. But most people should be able to choose one of the following routines and integrate it successfully into their daily lives. Remember that it won't be easy at first. Your mind is going to rebel and try to do everything in its power to keep you from concentrating. But with practice, perseverance, and the proper mental attitude, you should soon begin to find that meditation will work to relieve some of life's stressors.

Setting Up a Meditation Regime

No matter which type of meditation you choose, when starting out, try to meditate twice a day for at least 20, and ideally 30 minutes per session. If you find this exceedingly difficult, lower your sights and try an absolute minimum of 10 minutes per session during the first few weeks. When you're able to handle the 10-minute meditation session comfortably, gradually increase your time until you reach at least 20 minutes.

There is no ideal time during the day to meditate, although many find that the calmness of the early morning hours just after awakening is best. Others can interrupt their daily schedules just about any time to meditate. Still others find that meditation just before the evening meal is the right time. Others meditate just before bedtime, but beginners should be wary of this time because they are apt to fall asleep.

Unless it's terribly inconvenient, try meditating at first in the early morning and again following your evening meal—say at 6:30 in the morning and at 8:00 at night. But feel free to meditate any other time that you feel suits you.

As is the case with the physical relaxation exercises, choose a quiet, out-of-the-way place to meditate—somewhere where you won't be bothered by any outside interruptions. Wear loose clothing, and sit in a comfortable chair or on a well-padded rug.

It's essential to sit with your back straight but relaxed. You should place your hands unfolded in your lap or atop the arms of your chair. Some people prefer quiet classical music in the background while meditating, but most practitioners need total silence. Another option is to burn a candle or turn the lights off. Just don't sit in glaring direct light. You may wish to burn incense. Many yoga practitioners find that this practice eases their path toward meditation. It is entirely up to you. Never drink alcohol or use drugs prior to meditation. And don't meditate right after eating a large meal. It's a good idea to relieve yourself before meditation; you don't want any interruptions, even for the call of nature. The idea is to achieve total concentration with no distractions.

Now you're ready to begin. But not quite. Sit down. Center yourself. Take a few deep abdominal breaths. This is just to relax you initially. Do not breathe abdominally during your meditation. This can distract you from the task at hand. Breathe normally during meditation, and you'll soon find that your breathing will slow down. One thing you *can* do is try to observe your breathing during meditation. You can repeat your mantra in time with your inhalations and exhalations.

What about a mantra? Do you need one? Practitioners of certain types of meditation, such as Transcendental Meditation (TM) founded by Maharishi Mahesh Yogi, maintain that each person needs a specific mantra, a word or phrase in Sanskrit, the ancient Indian language, to be given personally by the guru or one of his disciples. The TM meditator is instructed never to divulge his mantra and never to repeat it except while meditating.

Other practitioners say that only words or phrases that have no meaning to the meditator achieve the desired results of meditation. They therefore advocate the use of a Sanskrit or other foreign language word or even a nonsense word in English as a mantra. Some yoga sects teach that the meditator should inwardly repeat a name of one of the Hindu gods or a phrase praising the gods in Sanskrit, such as the by now famous Hare Krishna chant.

Others concentrate on a series of sounds and their cadence and meter. Some yoga sects maintain that any Sanskrit word or phrase containing an *M* or *N* sound will do the trick. Still others argue that any word at all— whether it's in English or any other language—whether the meditator knows it or not, will, if repeated over and over, serve the goals of meditation. This repetition is the crucial ingredient that focuses the mind and brings about the meditative state.

We tend to agree with the last proposition. Psychological tests have borne out the fact that meditators can achieve the same mental and physical relaxation effects by repeating a Sanskrit word, an English word, or a nonsense word. So, we leave the choice of a mantra entirely up to you. You can sign up for a meditation course that includes a personalized mantra, or you can choose any word in any language. Here, to help you, is a list of words that have been used successfully by meditators.

> *One*
> *In* (while inhaling), *Out* (while exhaling)
> *Ocean*
> *Flower*
> *Garden*
> *Sail*
> *Rock*
> *Love*
> *Smooth*
> *Om* (pronounced "oh-m-m-m")
> *Ram* (pronounced "rahm")
> *Calm*
> *Rama* (pronounced "rah-maa")
> *Shanti* (pronounced "shan-tee," the Sanskrit word for peace)
> *Hare Om* (pronounced "hah-ray-ohm")
> *Om Nama Shivaya*
> *Nam Myoko Renge Kyo*

Once you've chosen a mantra, stick with it. That is, unless you find that repeating it keeps you from achieving the benefits of meditation. If that is the case, then by all means change it. But give your first choice a few days of use before abandoning it. And do not change—ever—during the middle of your meditation. Your mind will want to, but stay with your mantra for at least a few sessions before trading it in for another.

To begin meditating, simply repeat your mantra. The pace you choose is up to you. But err on the side of slowness. Stretch out a one-syllable mantra such as "one" or "om" into an elongated syllable, so that you can coordinate your repetitions with your breathing. Remember *not* to breathe too deeply; breathe normally. Coordinate your mantra repetitions with your breath. As you breathe in and out, repeat your mantra.

Inevitably, during meditation a thought will intrude. The best way to cope with outside thoughts is to complete them, then put them out of your mind, and concentrate on getting back to your mantra.

The best way to keep track of time when you're meditating is to keep a watch or clock nearby and glance at it when you think you've meditated for your allotted period of time. If you don't want to interrupt your meditative state, try using rosary beads as a counting and relaxing device. Some Hindu meditators use *japa mala*—a 109-bead device strung together on a string. The idea is to repeat one mantra for each bead. The one hundred ninth bead is larger than the others and is used to signal that you've reached one circuit. Using this type of rosary not only helps you count your mantras unobtrusively and without thinking about it, but also helps you remain alert in your meditation. Moreover, the action of fingering the beads also helps you repeat your mantra rhythmically and continuously.

When you're finished meditating, don't get up right away and go about your normal tasks. Sit still for a few minutes. Reflect on how you feel mentally and physically. Think about your upcoming activities, and try to carry over the calmness and sense of well-being you've achieved through meditation into your everyday activities. When you feel yourself in need of a relaxation break during the day, try a quick 5-minute meditation. The longer you meditate successfully, the better able you'll be to call upon the relaxing nature of meditation during instances of everyday stress.

1. Kenneth R. Pelletier, *Mind as Healer, Mind as Slaver* (Delta Books, 1977), pp. 193–94.

8 / Reducing Stress with Yoga

> Yoga has been one of the most successful methods of decreasing stress through a mixture of mental and physical approaches.
>
> Professor Jere E. Yates,
> *Managing Stress.*

One of the best ways to ease the muscular tension that stressors can bring is by practicing a series of ancient Indian stretching exercises called yoga. The yoga stretches—called poses or postures—also provide a very welcome side benefit: They help loosen the tight muscles that are responsible for cramps, strains, and pulls.

One of the basic tenets of yoga is proper relaxation. While you do the yoga exercises you also concentrate on relaxing. Yoga, therefore, provides both physical relaxation to the muscles and a meditative, calming relaxation to the mind.

As is the case with the other relaxation techniques, studies have shown that experienced yoga practitioners can lower their heart rates and blood pressure, and can increase the number of alpha waves to the brain—three proven countermeasures to the stressors of life. In addition, yoga practice can build muscle strength, especially in the back, as well as provide flexibility to all the major muscles. Finally, at the start, in between each exercise, and at the end of a yoga session come concentrated periods of relaxation which are very similar to the relaxation and autosuggestion techniques described in chapter 11.

Getting Started on a Yoga Routine

There are scores of instructional books on how to undertake a yoga regime. Among the best are *Introduction to Yoga* by Richard Hittleman (1969), *Integrated Yoga Hatha* by Swami Satchidananda (1970), and *The Complete Illustrated Book of Yoga* by Swami Vishnu Devananda (1972).

Another way to get started with yoga is to find a beginner's class at a health club or yoga center or at an adult education center. Or you can join an open class at a yoga center—one designed for beginners, intermediates, and advanced yoga students. As with all the other stress-reduction techniques discussed in this book, once you learn the basics of yoga, you can do an entire routine or a few postures of your choice any time during the day. One of the best things about yoga is that it requires no equipment or facilities not found in your home. All you need is a well-padded rug, a sheet or mat of some sort, and some loose exercise clothing, such as gym shorts and a T-shirt will do, or a T-shirt and light, billowing cotton yoga pants or a leotard. Never wear tight clothing such as blue jeans or shirts with buttons.

The best time of day to do your yoga routine is entirely up to you. For some, the quiet, early-morning hours are best. But others find their muscles are too stiff in the morning and they are unable to stretch out fully and properly. Some yoga centers offer midday yoga classes—

the perfect antidote to the three-martini (or wine or beer) lunch for working people.

Another good time of day for yoga is in the late afternoon, after the events of the day, but before the evening meal. A slow, calming, relaxing yoga session at that time can cut away the day's tensions, and contribute to a relaxing, productive evening.

If you're going to undertake a yoga routine on your own, here are some hints to help you get started. The yoga routine we suggest will take you about 45–60 minutes to complete. If you're in a big hurry, you can cut the routine to about half an hour. But always remember— even if you're in a hurry—never rush things when you're doing yoga. Take things slowly at all times during the routine. You can gain time if you're in a hurry by cutting down on the rest period between exercises or the time you hold each posture.

It's essential to breathe diaphragmatically during the entire yoga session. We discuss the basics of this type of deep breathing both in chapter 11 on relaxation exercises, and in a separate chapter on breathing itself.

But here's a mini-lesson in deep, diaphragmatic breathing. You do it through your nose with your mouth closed. The exhalations begin deep in the abdominal area, and the inhalations end there. As you exhale, your stomach draws in; as you inhale your stomach expands like a balloon.

Proper diaphragmatic breathing is a vital part of the yoga routine because it helps relax the body while also enabling you to stretch your muscles without undue discomfort. By concentrating on your breath during near-ly every moment of your yoga routine you help yourself relax, enable the muscles to stretch out, and become more flexible.

Try to keep your eyes closed during most of the yoga session. This will enable you to concentrate fully on what you are doing and will help shut out extraneous thoughts. Another important thing to keep in mind is never to try to do too much. Don't overstretch. Don't overstrain. Don't try to accomplish more than your body is capable of doing. Yoga exercises require effort, but you should never push yourself to the point where you overstretch. When you overstretch, the muscles tighten instead of relax, and you defeat the entire purpose of the yoga routine.

On the other hand, you should not baby yourself. To get all the benefits from yoga, you must work right up to the point of overstraining, but you should never exceed that point. There is an old adage in yoga: no pain, no gain. Keep that in mind. But also keep in mind that any pain you feel is a warning from the muscles that you are overstraining. When you feel the pain, ease up slightly. You should always be in control.

Since there is no competition in yoga, you do not have to adhere to any hard and fast rules on how long to hold individual postures. If we suggest holding a posture, say, for 4 minutes, and you feel very uncomfortable after 2 minutes, you owe it to yourself to loosen yourself from the posture and relax. This is true especially for beginners. But even experienced yoga practitioners sometimes have days when the body cannot handle a full routine. The most important thing is to stick with your yoga. Practice it regularly—at the very least 3 times a week—and before long you will begin to be rewarded.

Yoga to Reduce Stress

Here's a yoga routine designed especially to counterbalance the effects of stress on the mind and body. It is a basic hatha yoga routine that includes the major postures and emphasizes proper relaxation. There are dozens of variations on each basic posture. You can learn them (or

even invent variations of your own) once you've mastered
the basics and have become an experienced yoga practitioner.
The variations serve as a way of spicing up your yoga
sessions and presenting you with fresh challenges. But
beginners should first concentrate on mastering the basics.

Choose an area in your house with enough room for
you to stretch out fully in all directions. Keep your lights
dim; burn a candle or some incense if you wish. Don't play
music. It's important to have a serene, isolated atmosphere.
Don't eat anything heavy for 3 hours prior to a yoga
session. Keep a watch or clock nearby to time your exercises.

Spread out your sheet or blanket over the rug. This
helps save wear and tear on the rug, and also makes your
normal surrounding a little bit special to get you in the
mood for a special type of exercise.

To start the routine, sit with your eyes closed in a
comfortable, cross-legged position. Just try to relax, and
sit with your back straight. Take 1 or 2 deep, diaphragmatic
breaths, counting very slowly to 4 as you inhale, holding
your breath for 2 counts and then exhaling for 4 seconds.
Remember: With abdominal breathing your stomach expands as you inhale and deflates when you exhale.

Try taking about 5 or 6 of these deep, diaphragmatic
breaths. Try to visualize the air ebbing and flowing through
your body. This will help you block out all other thoughts.
After you've taken these 5 or so deep breaths, allow your
breathing to return to its normal rate. Then just sit still
and relax with your eyes closed for a minute or two. This
simple routine gets your mind and body ready to begin
the yoga exercises.

The first few exercises are warm-ups, rather than stretches.
Begin with neck rolls, the same ones we described on page
57. Go slowly, concentrating on your neck muscles only.
Do 8–10 rounds of the individual neck stretches and 3–5
complete rolls. You can do neck rolls, by the way, any time
during the day as an instant relaxation technique. If you

find yourself hunched over a desk, typewriter, or video terminal all day, or if you are involved in any sort of work in which you have to read a good deal, you can store a great deal of tension in the neck muscles, especially in the back of the neck. A daily diet of neck rolls when you're feeling particularly tense in that area can help ease the tension and make your neck muscles more flexible.

After you finish the neck rolls, just relax. Again, sit still with your eyes closed concentrating on your breath. The next warm-up exercises are the eye exercises, which stretch the eye muscles in a similar manner in which the neck rolls stretch the neck muscles. Eye exercises practiced regularly can help relieve eye strain problems caused by too much reading, concentration, or even television watching.

Here's how the yoga eye exercises work. Remain seated on the floor in your comfortable cross-legged position. Now open your eyes gently. Without moving your head, look toward the ceiling. Look as high as you can without overstraining, and hold the gaze up there for 2 seconds. Do not overstrain at any time. Then look down as far as you can toward the floor. Hold your gaze there for 2 seconds. Then look up.

Do the ceiling-to-floor routine for 10 rounds. Then close your eyes for a few seconds to let them relax. Now open your eyes and look to the right as far as possible without overstraining. Hold it for 2 seconds, and then move your gaze back to the center and then look all the way to the left, again without overstraining. Close your eyes again after 10 rounds of the right-to-left eye stretches.

When you open your eyes again, look as far as you can to the upper right. Hold the stretch there for 2 seconds, then shift the gaze to the lower left as far as you can see without overstraining. Repeat the upper-right-to-lower-left stretch for 10 rounds. Next do 10 rounds of stretching the eye muscles by looking first to the extreme upper left and then shifting to the extreme lower right. Then close your eyes for a few seconds.

Now do 5 very, very slow clockwise circles with the eyes, followed by 5 counterclockwise ones. Make sure you stretch the circles out as widely as possible without overstraining. After you've finished the full circles, close your eyes. Then rub your palms together vigorously until you feel them getting warm. Immediately cup your palms over your closed eyes and feel the soothing warmth seep in. Lightly massage your eyeballs with the tips of your fingers for a few seconds. Then relax.

The Sun Salutation

Now you're ready for the sun salutation, one of the best overall stretches for the entire body. Stand up slowly. Keep your eyes open at first until you get the hang of the sun salutation. Stand with your feet together, arms at your sides. Rotate your shoulders in a shrugging motion 2 or 3 times to loosen them up. Raise your arms to shoulder level, extend them, and slowly swing the arms from side to side. Don't move your feet. Now relax, and take a giant inhalation; hold your breath for a second and exhale slowly.

When you do the sun salutation, pretend you're a ballet dancer. Each movement should be smooth, effortless, and rhythmical. Concentrate only on what you are doing at each moment. Don't let your mind wander. Try to coordinate your breathing with the different steps of the exercise.

To start, exhale deeply and place your palms together in front of you at chest level, with your fingers pointing upward. Now inhale, lock your thumbs together and slowly raise your arms out in front of you as if you are pushing an object away from you. Just as you reach your full arm

extension, raise your arms to the ceiling, and then extend
them backward, arching your back and head until you feel
a good stretch. Keep your thumbs intertwined and your
arms alongside your ears. Your feet should be planted
firmly in place. Stretch back, but don't overstrain.

Now exhale and bring your arms back up toward the
ceiling, then stretch them out in front of you, keeping
your head between your arms. Then bend forward and
bring your palms to the floor on either side of your feet.
Bend your knees if you have to to get your palms flat on
the floor. Tuck your forehead into your knees. Don't
forget to breathe.

Keeping your palms on the floor and your left foot in
place, extend your right leg all the way back and balance
yourself on your right knee and right toes. Look up. Your
left foot should be where it was—between your hands.
Your left knee should touch your chest. Feel the stretch in
the quadricep muscles on the front of your extended right
leg and in the hamstrings in the back of your left leg.

Now extend your left leg back so that you are in the
push-up position. Try to keep your body straight. Don't
sag, and don't arch your back. Hold the push-up position
for a second or two, and then exhale deeply and drop
your knees to the floor, roll your chest down to the floor
between your hands and place your forehead on the floor
in front of your hands. Your rear end should be up in the
air.

Slide your chest forward while exhaling and go into the
cobra position with your stomach on the floor and your
chest and head arched backward. Keep your elbows bent
alongside your body. Look at the ceiling. You should feel
the muscles stretching out in your lower back. Hold the
pose for 2 seconds, and then exhale and move into the
inverted V position. You do this by pushing down with
your palms and coming up on your hands and toes. The
body should form an arch with your head between your

arms. Look back at your feet and try to bring your heels to the floor. Don't overstrain. Feel the tension in your hamstrings.

Without moving your hands or your left leg, bring your right foot up between your palms. Keep the left leg extended back and balance yourself on your left knee and toes. Your right leg should be thrust forward with the right foot between your hands. Keep your head up and back. Then exhale and bring your left leg forward so it is beside your right leg between your palms. Bend over and bring your head into your knees. Bend your knees if you have to.

Finally, inhale deeply and stretch forward with your arms, then straighten up and back and then relax by bringing your arms down to your sides. Take a deep abdominal breath, and then repeat the sun salutation at least 5 more times. Alternate thrusting your left and right legs each time.

After you've finished at least 6 sun salutations, lie on your back with your feet 18 inches apart and your arms away from your sides, palms up. This is one of the easiest, but also one of the most relaxing yoga postures. It is known as the corpse pose. As always during a yoga routine you should now begin to breathe deeply. Take this time also to roll your head from side to side, to shake out the tension in your legs and arms and to just plain relax. Relax and rest in the corpse pose without moving for another 3 minutes, until your breathing returns to its normal rate.

The Leg Lifts

Next come the leg-stretching exercises. We'll do the legs singly at first, and then work with both legs together. While you're doing these leg lifts, try to keep the rest of the body relaxed. Try especially hard not to tense up the muscles in your face, neck, or shoulders. Your natural inclination as you begin these leg lifts will be to scrunch up your face, so be aware of it, and try to relax. It will be difficult at first, but if you work on it, you should be able to relax completely and still do the leg-stretching exercises.

These exercises are done lying on your back. From the corpse pose, bring your legs together and place your arms alongside your body, palms up. Point your right heel toward the ceiling and your toes toward your head. Inhale, and slowly lift your right leg to a count of 5. Keep your left leg on the floor and keep it straight. Try not to move the left leg at all. Raise the right leg to 90 degrees if you can—again, don't overstrain—and then exhale and allow the leg to return very slowly to the floor. Do the same with your left leg. Keep breathing deeply as you do the leg lifts. Time your inhalations with your lifts, and exhale as you let your legs slowly down.

After you've done 2 or 3 individual leg lifts, it's time to limber up your ankles. So, inhale your right leg up as you did before. But this time, when you get to your maximum height, keep the leg up there and flex your ankle so that your big toe is pointed toward the ceiling. Hold your foot in that position for a second and then point the big toe back toward your head. Then point it up toward the ceiling again, and back toward the head once more. Follow this by flexing your ankle toward the left, then toward the right. Finally, make small circles with your ankle, going first in a clockwise direction and then counterclockwise. Remember to keep all the other muscles in the leg totally relaxed. Slowly lower your leg and repeat the ankle-flexing with the left leg.

For the final round of single leg lifts, raise your right leg, then reach up with your hands and grab the leg wherever you can get a hold of it. Ever so slowly and carefully, pull the leg toward you and at the same time, raise your forehead toward your knee. Keep breathing and don't overstrain. Hold the position for a few seconds, and then very slowly release the leg. Bring your arms back to your sides and slowly exhale the leg down. Repeat with the left leg.

Now relax in the corpse pose for at least 30 seconds before starting the double leg lifts. As with the single leg lifts, bring your legs together and your arms to your sides. Point both heels toward the ceiling and the toes back toward the head. Remembering to keep your upper body and face totally relaxed, inhale and slowly raise both legs as far as you can without overstraining. Keep the legs straight and keep them together.

Hold the legs at the apex of your stretch—90 degrees maximum—for a few seconds. Then slowly, with control, exhale and let your legs easily down to the floor. Try doing 10 double leg lifts. This will be hard to do at first because leg lifts require strong back and stomach muscles. If you cannot do 10 leg lifts at first, don't worry. Merely do as many as you can without overstraining. If you keep at it, you'll soon notice your back and stomach muscles gaining strength, and you'll be able to do more repetitions without too much trouble.

The Headstand

After the leg lifts comes what yoga teachers say is the most valuable exercise in the routine, the headstand. As is the case with so many other valuable things, it's very difficult for most people to do a headstand at first. It takes strong arm and back muscles, a sense of balance, and most of all, overcoming what can be a very powerful fear of falling.

Some beginners' yoga classes do not even attempt to teach the headstand. And if you feel that you do not wish

to try it, by all means skip this posture and go straight to
the next one, the shoulder stand. We include instructions
for the headstand here because it is such a good stretch
for the entire body and because some beginners may want
to attempt it.

To begin the headstand, slowly bring yourself from the
corpse pose up on your knees and into the child's pose.
Your forehead should be on the floor. Your arms should
be outstretched behind you alongside your body, palms
up. Your chest is folded on top of your knees.

Relax in the child's pose for at least 20 seconds. Then sit
up on your heels. Fold your arms across your chest and
fall forward slowly, catching yourself on the floor with
your arms. The object is to make an equilateral triangle
with your forearms. To do so simply grab your elbows
with the opposite hands. Make sure you're touching the
same part of your elbows with the hands. Once you've
measured off the equal distance, keep your elbows on the
floor in the same spot. Don't move them. With your elbows
in place on the floor, extend your forearms forward to
form the top angle of the triangle. Interlace your fingers
to form a cup with your hands. Place the crown of your
head on the floor. The back of your head should be
supported by your locked fingers. Extend your thumbs up
alongside the back of your neck for balance.

Now arch your back by coming up on your toes, so that
your rear end is up in the air. Very slowly and carefully
tiptoe forward, keeping your back arched until you reach
the point where you can feel yourself balancing on your
arms. Tuck your knees into your chest and balance on
your arms. Beginners should go no further. Just stay in
this position so you can feel where the balance is that
you'll need for the full headstand. Hold the position as
long as you can without overstraining, a maximum of 5
minutes. Then relax slowly by first letting your legs slowly
and gently hit the floor and folding yourself back into the

child's pose once again. If you cannot feel the balance, or if your back or arms cannot support your weight, *do not* try the headstand. Instead, go directly to the shoulder stand. After you've worked at the shoulder stand, you may want to come back again and try the headstand.

If you find that you can do the preliminary parts of the headstand without undue pain or strain after practicing for a week or so, you should be ready to try the full headstand. From the point where you're balancing on your forearms, all you do is slowly raise both legs, keeping the knees bent. Slowly lift your thighs so that they're parallel to the floor, but keep the knees still tucked in. Finally, straighten the thighs up slowly and inch your way carefully into an erect full headstand.

Here are a couple of things to keep in mind about the headstand. Breathe deeply the whole time you hold the pose. It helps the body relax, and also brings fresh air deeply into the lungs. Try to push down with your arms and keep very little weight on your head while you're in the position. Since you're really supporting yourself mostly with your arms, the headstand actually might be called an arm stand. The arms should be doing most of the work. When you feel tired—and for most beginners, this should happen after you're in the full headstand for about a minute—come down very slowly and with control. Bend your legs at the knee, fold them into your chest, and slowly uncurl down. Keep your head on the floor even after you've come down. Without moving your head off the floor, immediately go into the child's pose for at least a minute. This will give your system time to recuperate fully from the inverted position of the headstand.

From the child's pose, slowly get back to the corpse pose. Breathe deeply for a few seconds. Don't forget to keep your eyes closed. Then just relax. Feel the effects of the headstand. Yoga teachers say the headstand is the "king" of the yoga postures because the body derives so many benefits from it. If you stay in the position for at least 5 minutes, the blood circulates through your system completely while you are inverted. You can certainly feel the blood "going to your head" while you're in the headstand. And your face should turn a shade redder if you keep holding the pose for 5 minutes.

Best of all, the headstand, as is the case with other inverted postures such as the shoulder stand, gets pressure and tension off your feet and legs, something that few of us do during the day. Even when we sit, we exert pressure on our lower extremities. Getting them up in the air even for a few minutes provides a countermeasure to the pressures each of us places on the feet and legs every day.

The Shoulder Stand

You can get many of these benefits from the shoulder stand. And it's much easier to do—so easy that all beginners should be able to do the posture without too much trouble. If you've just finished the headstand, relax in the corpse pose for at least 5 minutes. To get into the shoulder stand, start, as always, from the corpse pose. Bring your hands, palms down, alongside your body. Keeping your legs together, inhale and bring them slowly up to a 90-degree position. Now roll your trunk into a vertical position, sliding your hands behind your back for support. Keep your elbows on the floor. Your thumbs should be pressing into your sides and your other fingers should be extended up on your back just above the buttocks. While in the shoulder stand, the back of your neck should be flat on the ground, and your chin should be pressed into your chest.

The shoulder stand will feel uncomfortable at first. But try to relax into the position anyway. The best way to do this is to breathe deeply and to concentrate on what you are doing with your body. Picture your legs extended straight as you keep your eyes closed and breathe deeply.

Try to hold the shoulder stand at first for 60 seconds. If you feel tired, instead of coming completely out of the position, try resting your knees on your forehead. But remember not to push yourself too hard, and don't overstrain. Try holding the position a few seconds longer each time you practice it. The ultimate goal is to stay in the shoulder stand for 10 minutes.

The shoulder stand has many benefits. It helps strengthen the back muscles, brings relaxation and flexibility to the feet and legs, and reputedly helps regulate the thyroid gland, which is located at the base of the neck.

It's very important to take your time unfolding from the shoulder stand. Roll out of the position in reverse order compared to the way in which you went up. Remember to exhale as you unfold and to keep control of your body at all times. It's also vital to keep your head riveted on the floor at all times as you're coming out of the shoulder stand. Don't jerk it off the floor when you roll down. After you've come down from the shoulder stand, immediately assume the corpse pose. Since you've just put pressure on your neck, do a few stretches to relieve any tension that remains in that area. Roll your head from side to side a few times, breathing deeply all the while.

The Fish Pose

Stay in the corpse pose for at least 2 or 3 minutes to recuperate from the shoulder stand. Remain motionless, concentrating only on your breath. The next pose, which is called the fish position, stretches the neck in the opposite direction and is considered the counter pose to the shoulder stand. After resting for about 2 minutes in the corpse pose, go into the fish pose by putting your arms beneath your body so that your palms are under your thighs. Arch your back, supporting yourself with both elbows. Try to put the crown of your head on the floor. Even though your head is on the floor, you should be supporting nearly all of your body weight with your elbows. As always, breathe deeply.

This pose probably will feel awkward at first. If you feel dizzy, try breathing even more deeply. If this doesn't cure the dizziness, slowly come down into the corpse pose and breathe deeply. Try the fish again, but if you continue getting dizzy, quit immediately.

It's best to hold the fish pose for the same amount of time you held the shoulder stand. But, as is the case with all the yoga positions, how long you hold the position is entirely up to you. Go at your own pace. Listen to your body. Don't baby yourself, but don't overstrain either.

To get yourself out of the pose, keep supporting your body with your elbows and raise your head off the floor, placing it down very slowly and gently. Then bring your arms out from under your body and assume the corpse pose. Begin relaxing your entire body by taking 3 or 4 deep, diaphragmatic breaths and then letting your breathing return to normal.

To help yourself relax after the fish pose, roll your head from side to side several times in the corpse pose. Bounce your legs gently up and down. Shake out your hands. Since you've been tensing up your neck, try to relax it in this manner: Interlace your fingers behind your head, and using only your arms, pull your head gently off the floor and pull it toward your chest. Don't overstrain. These muscles are delicate. Be very careful. Hold the head in the forward position for a few seconds and then slowly and carefully stretch it to the left and then back to the center and then over to the right. Pull it toward the center again, then toward the chest once more, and then let your head go slowly back to the floor. Roll the head again from side to side one last time then relax completely.

The Forward-Bending Pose

Rest in the corpse pose for a good 3 or 4 minutes, concentrating on nothing but relaxing and following your breath as you inhale and exhale normally. The next group of postures, the forward bends, stretch out the back and leg muscles. To get ready for the forward-bending poses, bring your legs together and stretch your arms out over your head while you're lying on the floor. Now give both arms and legs a good, long gentle stretch. Stretch out as far as you can comfortably. Then release all the tension and relax. Now stretch your left arm and left leg. Relax. Then stretch the right arm and right leg. Relax. Then stretch the left arm and right leg, then the right arm and left leg. Relax. Finally, give all four a good stretch, pull in the muscles of your stomach, hold it for a few seconds, and then relax.

Now stretch your arms over your head and sit up all in one motion. Keep your arms outstretched toward the ceiling as you sit up. Your legs should be straight and together out in front of you. Inhale and stretch your arms up. Exhale and bend forward, stretching your entire body out over your legs. Try to touch your toes. Don't worry if you can reach only your knees or ankles. With practice, you'll be able to get more flexibility. Remembering to keep breathing, hold the forward bend at the position you can reach easily for a minute. Don't overstrain, and don't bounce. Find the position where you're bending forward and stretching out to your maximum level without overdoing it. Hold that position.

After a minute, take a big inhalation and slowly raise

your arms back up over your head. Bounce your legs up and down to get rid of some of the tension. Roll your legs a bit to the left and right. Now try a variation—with your left leg extended, place your right foot on top of your left thigh. Place your hands on your right knee and gently bounce the leg up and down. Then place the right foot on the floor and tuck it into the inside of your left thigh. Reach up with both hands and exhale down over your extended left leg. Again, come to rest wherever you feel comfortable. Hold the pose for 30 seconds, and then slowly release, relax, and come up. Repeat with the right leg extended and the left leg hooked next to the right inner thigh near the groin.

The Inclined Plane

Now try one more forward bend with both legs extended out in front of you. This time, you should be able to come down a tiny bit further than you did initially. After a minute's stretch, come up. Now drop your arms behind your back to get ready to move into the next position, the inclined plane. This is done with the palms down behind your back, fingers facing away from you. The hands should be positioned at about shoulder width. Support yourself with your arms, and slowly raise your body off the floor. The aim is to get the body into a straight line.

Once again, this is a position which will feel uncomfortable at first, but try it anyway. Hold the inclined plane for about 15–20 seconds. Then slowly come out of the position by simply sitting down slowly. Lie back down on your back, assuming the corpse pose once again. Roll your head from side to side and shake out any tension in the arms and legs.

The Backward-Bending Poses

Rest in the corpse pose for at least a minute before going into the first backward-bending pose. The backward bends complement the forward bends. A full yoga routine consists of three backward postures—the cobra, locust, and bow. But, if you are pressed for time, you need do only one, preferably the bow, because it gives a more complete stretch to the back muscles and the spine.

There is a special relaxation pose to get you ready for the backward bends. To get there, roll over on your stomach and make a pillow with your hands by placing one palm atop the other. Then rest your cheek on top of the top hand. Use either cheek and face in either direction. Your big toes should be touching, and your feet should fall out to the sides. Stay in this extremely relaxing position for about a minute. Don't forget to breathe comfortably.

The first backward bend is the cobra. Visualize a cobra snake as you prepare to emulate it. From the relaxation pose, bring your legs together and point your toes into the floor. Put your forehead on the floor. Place your palms under your shoulders, and slide slowly up into the position, like a cobra uncoiling. Keep your legs together. Slowly brush your forehead, then your nose, and finally your chin along the floor. Then bring up the head and look toward the ceiling as you push down with your hands. Slowly come up, breathing all the while, until you reach a point where your elbows are bent about halfway. Hold the elbows in toward the body, and hold the cobra for about 20 seconds.

The cobra is not a push-up. Your stomach, abdomen, and legs should remain on the floor the entire time. Your elbows should be bent. Breathe deeply while you're in the cobra and when you feel tired, roll yourself slowly down. Do 2 more cobras. When you finish the third, go into the special backward-bending relaxation posture, putting the opposite cheek on top of your hands.

The next back pose is the locust. It's a very demanding one, so rest for at least a minute after the cobra. And be very careful with the locust. Begin by placing your chin on the floor and bringing your arms alongside your body with the palms down. Keep your chin right there on the floor; inhale and lift your left leg up as high as you can. Don't swivel your hips. Don't move the right leg. Concentrate only on the leg that's up in the air. Hold the left leg up there for about 10 seconds, and then slowly release the leg and bring it gently to the floor. Do the same thing with the right leg, then repeat once more with the left and again with the right leg.

Now you're ready for the full locust pose. Keep your chin on the floor, make fists with both hands, and put your arms under your body this time. The fists should be under the thighs. Take 3 deep breaths. On the third inhalation, lift both legs into the air as high as you can. Hold them there for as long as you can—aim for about 10 seconds at first. Then relax, bring your legs down, and assume the backward-bending relaxation pose for at least a minute.

The final back pose is the bow. To do this, put your forehead on the floor, reach back, and grab your feet. Pull them slowly backward toward your head to stretch the legs. Then grab your ankles, inhale, and slowly lift your head, chest, and thighs, and at the same time arch your back and lift up both legs. Balance on your stomach for about 15 seconds, then exhale and bring your forehead back to the floor and drop your thighs. Keep hold of your ankles. Then rest for a few seconds. Then inhale and do one more bow. Hold it for about 20 seconds before coming down. On your third bow, once you've balanced on your stomach, rock back and forth 6–10 times. This gives an extra stretch to the entire body and also provides a light massage to the internal organs. You deserve a rest after the rocking bow. Collapse into the relaxation position and breathe and relax for 2 or 3 minutes.

Now slowly bring yourself into the child's pose to further relax the back muscles. To get into the child's pose from the relaxation position, just place your hands under your shoulders and come up on your knees. Keep your hands extended on the floor for a preliminary stretch, and then sit back on your heels, putting your forehead on the floor. Let the backs of your arms fall limply to the floor at your sides. Hold the child's pose for a minute. It's a very relaxing position, and you can use it any time during the day as a quick relaxer. It's especially good for soothing the effects of menstrual cramps.

The Spinal Twist

The final position in the yoga routine is a spinal twist. You get there from the child's pose by sitting up on your ankles and shifting your body first to the right of your legs. Put your left leg over the right knee, with the sole of the foot flat on the floor. Your left knee should be close to your chest.

Slowly twist your body around to the left and raise your right arm above your head. Reach down and grab your left ankle with your right hand on the outside of your left foot. Twist your shoulders and head toward the left. Support yourself with your left hand extended on the floor behind your back. It's difficult to get into this contorted position at first. But if you take your time and relax, you should get the hang of it pretty quickly. You'll find that the position helps align your spine and relaxes the entire body.

Hold the spinal twist for at least 30 seconds. Then try it again on the other side for another 30 seconds. When you're finished, untangle yourself and just sit still on the floor. Then slowly stand up and stretch your arms first toward the ceiling and then let them fall loosely to the floor in front of you. Just hang there for 15 seconds or so and repeat the up-and-down stretches.

Do a few side stretches. With your feet planted at shoulder width and with your left arm at your left side and your right arm up and against your right ear, bend all the way to the left. Hold the stretch for a few seconds, and then come back to the center. Change arms, bend to the right, and hold. Relax and repeat several times.

Now we have reached the very last part of the routine: final relaxation. Get back down into the corpse pose. Roll your head from side to side several times. Stretch out your legs and arms and then relax them. Breathe deeply. Take 6 to 8 deep abdominal breaths. Spend the next 5–10 minutes practicing a mini-version of the relaxation autosuggestion technique we explain in chapter 6.

After the final relaxation, sit up slowly and carefully. Keep your eyes closed and remain seated in a comfortable cross-legged position. Feel what you've accomplished. Your muscles should be relaxed, flexible, and refreshed. Your mind should also be very relaxed and refreshed.

9/ Exercising to Relieve Stress

Regular exercise is one of the best methods of relieving stress.

Arthur Fisher, *The Healthy Heart.*

Doctors have known for quite some time that one of the very best ways to combat the effects of the stressful lifestyle is to undertake a regular, balanced exercise regime. Exercise to combat stress? It isn't as farfetched as you might think.

Sure, the main purpose of exercise is to get yourself into better physical condition. But there are a number of important things that exercising accomplishes to help minimize the harmful effects of stress.

Dr. Hans Selye, the pioneering stress researcher, suggests that one way to escape the pressures of daily life is to engage in some form of vigorous physical activity. When you engage in physical activity, according to Dr. Selye, you shut off the pressures of life by putting stress on the muscles instead.

Jim Fixx, the running guru, gives us an example of how this theory works in his popular book, *The Complete Book of Running*. "Suppose you work in an office and you come home tired, washed out, your energy gone," Fixx writes. "You dread the thought of running; yet as soon as you start, you feel better, and by the end of half an hour, you are restored. You may have felt tired, but you'll find to your surprise that you weren't tired at all. It's a pleasant discovery."[1]

There are other reasons why taking part in a regular exercise regime can help us overcome the effects of stress. For one thing, a well-rounded program of aerobic exercises and flexibility (stretching) exercises can help alleviate such physical stress reactions as increased blood pressure, an elevated heart rate, and muscle tension.

Aerobic exercises are the key to any exercise regime designed to mitigate the effects of stress. These are low-intensity, repetitive routines such as running, walking, cycling, swimming, and dancing. There has been an explosion of interest in aerobics in the last decade.

Importance of Aerobic Exercises

At the start of just about every "Alive and Well" program we take time to go through an aerobics routine. The reason is that aerobics, when done properly, not only make the cardiovascular system work more efficiently, but also help you lose excessive weight and provide you with a tangible sense of physical and mental well-being. When integrated into a balanced exercise regime—along with stretching and strength-building exercises—aerobics provides the key toward fighting off the harmful consequences of the stressful life-style.

The basic aerobic concept was developed by Dr. Kenneth Cooper in the mid-1960s. Since then, aerobic exercise regimes have been taken up by millions of Americans of both sexes, regardless of age or life-style. The basic aerobic theory is simple. It involves the heart and the heart's main job, pumping fresh blood into the muscles. Cooper found out that exercises that get the heart beating at 70–85 percent of its capacity for at least 20 consecutive minutes 3 times a week will increase the heart's efficiency. Aerobic exercises do for the heart's "muscles" what lifting weights does for the skeletal muscles. Aerobics make the heart muscles stronger, enabling them to work at maximum capacity with minimal exertion.

The proof that aerobics help your cardiovascular system perform more efficiently is that after about 6 months of proper aerobic training, your resting heartbeat will decrease. A lowered heartbeat means that the heart is doing its job, but that it is doing it without overexerting itself. Although we do not know whether the heart has a finite number of beats, it makes sense that the fewer times it beats the longer it will last.

What good does a lowered heartbeat do? Simply this: Those with efficient cardiovascular systems (and low heart rates) such as marathon runners, can run for long periods of time without undue fatigue. This is because their cardiovascular systems are operating at peak efficiency, delivering large volumes of fresh blood throughout their bodies rapidly as they call on their muscles to perform.

If you practice an aerobics routine faithfully for a few months, you will find that you will feel less tired during the day. You should be alert and feel strong physically and mentally even at the end of the longest, hardest working day. Just knowing that your body and mind are well conditioned can give you a feeling of confidence and well-being. This will make it easier for you to ward off the negative effects of the bombardment of stressors inherent in everyday life.

Before you begin an aerobics program, keep these things in mind. First, if you are over 30, it's best to take a physical examination before embarking on any type of exercise program. This is particularly true for those who have been physically inactive for long periods of time and live a sedentary life-style. Tell your doctor what type of exercise you're about to undertake and ask for specific advice. If you're over 35, it's wise to take a physical exam and make sure it includes a stress test. This is a treadmill test designed to see if you have any heart irregularities.

Another word of warning. Once you begin exercising, listen to your body. If you feel pain anywhere, if you get dizzy or feel nauseous, stop what you are doing *immediately* and relax. If the problem disappears, wait a few minutes and then start exercising again, but slowly. But be on the lookout. If the problem recurs, call it a day. If you continue exercising, you risk permanently damaging your body. If the pain recurs the next time you're exercising, it's best to check with your doctor before proceeding any further.

In aerobics you are concerned primarily with the amount of *time* you exercise, not the distance you cover. The main goal is to get your heartbeat going at 70–85 percent of its capacity. This figure is known as the target zone. If you don't get your heartbeat into the target zone, you won't be able to get the cardiovascular benefits of aerobics. If you go over your target zone, you risk damaging your heart.

The target zone figures are calculated by age. Find yours on the following chart:

Women		Men	
AGE	TARGET ZONE	AGE	TARGET ZONE
25	130–157	25	140–170
30	126–153	30	136–165
35	123–149	35	132–160
40	119–145	40	128–155
45	116–140	45	124–150
50	112–136	50	119–145
55	109–132	55	115–140
60	105–128	60	111–135
65	102–123	65	109–132

These figures are based on calculations derived from maximum heart rates based on age. But these heart rates vary slightly from person to person. If you have any doubt about your own maximum heart rate, or if you have any history of heart problems, be sure to check with your doctor to find out what heart rate you should shoot for during your aerobic exercising.

In order to find out if your heartbeat is in the target zone during aerobics, you have to learn to take your pulse. For this, you need a watch or clock with a sweep second hand. The best pulse point to use during exercise is either of the two carotid arteries found on the sides of your neck. To take your pulse using the carotid artery, just place your thumb in the middle of your chin and press the other four fingers into your throat gently on the side of your neck. Count the beats for 10 seconds, then multiply the number by 6 to get a close approximation of your heartbeat.

When you begin an aerobics routine, check your pulse several times just to get in the habit of doing it. Take your pulse just after you've warmed up, but before you set out on your exercises. Use this for comparison later. Then a few minutes after you've started your aerobic activity, take your pulse again while you are on the go. This will give you some idea of whether you are pushing yourself hard enough, or too hard. The most important time to take your pulse is immediately after you finish your aerobic routine. It's important to time your pulse just as you finish, since your pulse will descend rapidly once you stop.

After a few weeks' practice, you should be able to tell when you are in the target zone, when you're above it and should slow down, and when you're below it and should pick up your pace. Don't worry about not being able to get to the target zone for the first few weeks of your aerobic activity, especially if you haven't exercised for a while. You'll get there. Don't rush things.

The most important thing is to stick with your routine. Try keeping track of your progress in a written diary. Mark down your pulse rate before, during, and after aerobics, how long you were able to go without stopping, and how you felt before and after exercising. Even experienced aerobic exercisers should remember to check their heart rate every so often. Sometimes you can fall into patterns without realizing that you are either pushing yourself too hard, or not pushing yourself hard enough. So, experienced runners, walkers, swimmers, dancers, and other aerobic practitioners should check their pulse immediately upon stopping every month or so to make sure that they are in their target zone.

If you keep up a regular aerobics routine at least 3 times per week for 20–30 minutes of target-zone activity per session, you will begin to experience what Dr. Cooper calls the training effect. Basically, this means you are improving your cardiovascular system. Your heart and lungs will be working efficiently, and you will be able to exercise for longer periods of time without becoming overly tired. A clear signal that the training effect is happening occurs when your resting heartbeat lowers—perhaps as much as 5–10 beats per minute after 6 months to a year of steady aerobic activity.

Choosing the Best Type of Aerobic Exercise

Many different types of exercises provide aerobic benefits. These include dancing, running, walking, swimming, cycling, rope skipping, cross-country skiing, running in place, canoeing, sculling, working a rowing machine, nonstop calisthenics, handball, squash, basketball, and any other activity that involves continuous but not necessarily vigorous movement.

The type of aerobic activity that you choose, of course, is entirely up to you. But there are some criteria to keep in mind before you decide on one. The most important thing is how much time you have to spend on aerobics. Some of the routines require you to report to a gym, exercise club, or health spa to join in a group activity or use special equipment. If you can spare 45 minutes to an hour at least 3 times a week, then an aerobic routine such as dancing or swimming just may suit you. You'll have to search out a dancing class or swimming pool where lanes are reserved for exercise, but if you can spare the time, these two exercises might be for you.

The aerobic exercises that take up the least amount of time are running, walking, and bicycling. All you have to do to take part in these exercises is step out your front door and get on with it. If time is a crucial factor, we suggest that you go with one of these exercises.

Another important criterion in choosing an aerobic routine is what physical shape you're in. All of the aerobic exercises provide the same cardiovascular benefits, but some of them require much more vigorous exertion than others. Cross-country skiing, basketball, squash, and handball, for example, are exercises that sedentary persons should be leery of. These are very taxing undertakings, and to get aerobic benefit from them you must keep at them constantly. It is therefore best for those who haven't exercised for a while to stick with the less physically demanding routines: walking, running, cycling, dancing, or swimming.

Another thing to keep in mind in choosing a routine is that some are impractical to practice on a regular, year-round basis. You can't very well cross-country ski 12 months out of the year in most areas of North America, nor can you paddle a canoe all-year-round.

One final thing. Choose a regime that you'll enjoy doing. It's going to be hard enough, especially in the beginning, for you to keep to your exercising. Don't make things harder by choosing an exercise that you can't stand taking part in. Some aerobic exercises are just plain boring. Stay away from these—running in place, chair stepping, indoor cycling, and rowing—or you run the risk of getting soured very quickly and quitting.

Before we present some hints on how to get started on some recommended routines, let's go over some physical activities that are *not* aerobics. Golf, tennis, softball, touch football, and volleyball are all popular, enjoyable sports. They can also provide you with a way to run around and forget your troubles and tensions. For that reason, by all means feel free to take part in them. They'll help you deal with stressors by taking your mind off your problems, if only for a few hours. But these sports do not provide any aerobic benefits since they do nothing to increase your cardiovascular capacity.

Aerobic Dancing

Hundreds of thousands of women all over the country—and some men too—have found that aerobic dancing not only helps them look and feel better, but also is just plain fun. That's the extraordinary thing about aerobic dancing, sometimes called jazzercise. The enthusiastic claims made by aerobic dancers are true: If you follow a regular aerobic-dancing routine, you'll get the same cardiovascular benefits that you can derive from running, cycling, or swimming and you'll be strengthening and toning the muscles of your body. Best of all, you'll have a great time doing it.

Ever since the concept of aerobic dancing was developed in 1969 by Jacki Sorensen, classes have sprung up from coast to coast. The best way for a beginner to get involved is to sign up for such a class. Do some comparison shopping before you choose a class, however. Look in on one session to see if you feel comfortable with the surroundings. Ask class members if they're satisfied with the course. Once you sign up, be sure to tell the instructor that you're a beginner. A competent teacher will take extra time with you in the beginning to make sure that you don't overdo it and that you get the proper cardiovascular conditioning.

If you want to undertake an aerobic dancing routine on your own, here's what to do. First, find a room where you'll be able to dance around without hitting any furniture or walls. Make sure it's a place where you can play loud music without disturbing anyone. Also, be sure that the floor surface can take the pounding you'll be giving it. Don't do aerobic dancing on an expensive rug, and don't do it on a hard concrete floor. Find a carpeted area that you can abuse a bit.

You'll need a good pair of running shoes—or a special pair of aerobic dancing shoes now on the market—to protect your feet and legs. Next, pick out some music. Rock 'n' roll and disco are the best. Remember to choose at least 30 consecutive minutes of music. You also have the option of purchasing one of the many aerobic-dancing records available which provide hints and instructions in addition to bouncy rock music.

After you've chosen your music, it's time to get an idea of what type of movements you want to do during your aerobic-dancing routine. The object is to keep moving the entire time, but exactly how you move is entirely up to you. You can start by simply shuffling your feet in time to the music. After a few minutes, swing your arms around a bit and start running gently in place. Try kicking your knees up high in time to the beat, or use any other type of dance step you can think of. Just remember: It's essential to keep moving at all times. You can vary the intensity by slowing down, but don't stop moving altogether because your heartbeat will plummet, and you will lose any aerobic benefit.

Beginners should not attempt to dance continuously for the full 20 minutes for the first few weeks of aerobic dancing. Instead, beginners should aim to dance steadily for 5–10 minutes in these initial sessions. Always keep alert to the body's warning signals. If you feel shortness of breath or dizziness, stop immediately. Sit down and rest until you feel better. Try dancing again, but stop as soon as the warning signs reappear. Beginners should monitor their pulse regularly until they get a feel for how much effort they have to put into their dancing to get to the target zone. Remember: *Never* exceed your maximum target zone pulse.

Before you begin each aerobic-dancing session, it's a good idea to do about 5–10 minutes of stretching exercises. These serve three purposes: They get the muscles ready to perform the work needed during aerobics without undue strain; they help give your muscles flexibility; and they help you and your muscles relax.

You use your leg muscles extensively during aerobic dancing, so don't forget to pay particular attention to stretching the leg muscles before you begin. A good stretch emphasizing the leg muscles is the yoga sun salutation described on p. 77. Try doing 6–8 sun salutations very slowly but smoothly before your dancing routine. There are any number of other leg stretches you can do aside from the sun salutation. These include:

• A toe-touching stretch in which you stand with your feet about shoulder width apart and simply bend forward from the hips with your knees slightly bent, letting your hands fall toward the floor. Hang there for 15–20 seconds. Don't bounce. Feel your lower back, hips, groin, and hamstrings stretch out. Breathe evenly. Slowly come up and relax.

• To stretch the muscles in the front of the leg, stand

facing a wall and support yourself with your right hand. Reach back and grab your left foot with your left hand. Pull your left leg up until you feel the stretch on top of your thigh and calf. Hold it there without overstraining or bouncing for 20–30 seconds. Then release and switch legs.

• For an entire body elongation stretch, lie on your back on the floor with your feet extended out straight and together and your arms extended out over your head. Gently reach out with your arms and your legs until you feel a good, gentle total body stretch. Hold for 15–20 seconds and then release. Repeat twice. For an extra stretch, pull the stomach muscles in while stretching the arms and legs in this position.

One place to find many other good stretches is a book called *Stretching* by Bob Anderson. This book clearly shows you how to stretch out to prepare for all types of exercises.

After you've stretched out, you are ready to begin dancing. But don't go at it whole hog first. Take the first 5 minutes very slowly. Consider it part of your warm-up. Your muscles still aren't ready for a vigorous workout, but 5 minutes of warm-up dancing should do the trick.

A word of advice about intensity. Remember this is aerobic dancing, not the Olympics. You are not trying to break any world records. You are not trying to go as fast as you can. You're not competing with anyone. You're aiming for constant movement, just enough to get your heartbeat into that target zone for 15–20 minutes. So slow down, take it easy, and enjoy yourself. You may be surprised to find that you don't have to dance very vigorously to get your heart into the target zone.

Once you've finished your 15–20 minutes in the target zone you need to dance very slowly for another few minutes to wind down. Don't just stop. You've got to give the muscles time to cool down. So just move around very easily and slowly for the final 5 minutes of dancing. Then take 5 more minutes to do some light stretching or calisthenics. Use the same stretches you tried before you began dancing and add some leg lifts, side stretches, and sit-ups if you feel up to it. This postroutine stretching will prevent soreness and stiffness later on.

To get aerobic benefits from dancing, you should do your routine at least 3 times a week. Don't let more than 2 days go by between sessions. If you do, you'll lose aerobic benefits.

Walking

It may be difficult to believe, but you can get the same cardiovascular benefits from walking that you can from running or from any other aerobic exercise. Remember, aerobic walking is a bit more than strolling around the block. You have to walk fairly rapidly. Still, walking is the least strenuous of all the aerobic routines.

Another good thing about aerobic walking is that it is not repetitive. You get to go places while you walk, and you get a chance to observe what's around you. You can walk through parks and enjoy trees and flowers, or you can walk through downtown areas of cities and do a little window-shopping or people watching.

Walking is a good exercise for those with leg problems such as shin splints, or heel, ankle, knee, or other running-induced leg injuries. These leg problems are sure to bother you if you run, but they shouldn't present much of a problem if you undertake an aerobic-walking program. Walking also is good for overweight persons because of all the aerobic exercises, it puts the lightest demand on the cardiovascular system.

All you need in the way of equipment to start an aerobic-walking regime is a good pair of running shoes and loose-fitting, comfortable clothes. Any type of sturdy running shoe with a built-up heel will do for walking. Don't wear tennis shoes, though. They don't provide enough protection for the heel or instep.

To get aerobic benefits from walking, you've got to walk at a pretty brisk pace. You'll want to walk along at about a 15-minute-per-mile pace. Beginners probably will have a hard time keeping this pace. That's to be expected. The answer—as it is in all aerobic routines—is to start out very slowly without doing more than your muscles and cardiovascular system can handle. Then, after a few weeks, your cardiovascular capacity will improve and you can increase the intensity of your walking pace. With a few months' practice, you should be able to walk that 15-minutes-per-mile with ease.

As with all aerobic exercises, in walking you're not concerned with how many miles you cover each time you exercise. The only criterion is how much time you spend in the target zone. So, in walking, measure your pulse as you start out; check it again after you've been at it awhile. Soon, you'll be able to judge for yourself whether you need to step up your pace or cut it back to stay within your target zone.

Before beginning your routine, you need to stretch out those leg muscles. Take 5–10 minutes to do some yoga sun salutations or the leg stretches we describe on pp. 77 and 79. Then start walking slowly to warm up for 5 minutes. Then get into your aerobic walking pace for 20 minutes. End the routine with 5 minutes of very slow walking and another 5 minutes of leg stretches or calisthenics.

Here are some things to keep in mind about your aerobic-walking routine. You should have no pain whatsoever while you're walking. If you feel pain, it is a sign from your body telling you to let up. Listen to your body. Secondly, if you're walking at the correct pace, you should be able to carry on a conversation with someone alongside you easily. If you're panting and too winded to talk, you're pushing yourself too hard. Slow up. Finally, you should feel refreshed and not overly tired after you walk. If you are totally exhausted, you've pushed yourself too much. Next session, cut back on your intensity.

Exercise therapists believe that walking probably is the most relaxing and stress-easing of the aerobic routines. This is probably true because the walking pace allows you to drink in the serenity of a park on a beautiful day, for example, something that a swimmer, say, cannot do while exercising. Walking puts no drastic stress on any part of the body or mind. Maybe this fact more than anything else helps explain why walking is such a good antidote to the stress of everyday life.

Running

Running today is the "sexiest" aerobic exercise, probably because it's the most visible. Everywhere you go in this nation, you see men and women of all ages, sizes, and shapes out there pounding the pavement. Marathon races are now huge media events, and you can even buy designer running clothes—from designer socks to designer sweatbands.

Running appears to be an uncomplicated enough activity. But dozens of books have been written explaining the whys and wherefores of running. We present here some tips on getting the most from an aerobic-running routine while at the same time keeping in mind that our very important secondary objective in running is to mitigate the effects of stress.

The most important thing to keep in mind about running is that it can be dangerous. As we discussed on p. 110, this is not an activity that any physically inactive person should take lightly—especially if you are over 35 or overweight.

Once you've received permission from your doctor, you should still be extremely careful while running, especially during the first few weeks. Running greatly taxes the delicate cardiovascular system and requires strong leg muscles. This is why you must remember to start out very slowly, proceed extremely cautiously, and exert yourself more fully only after you're confident that your body can handle the extra exertion.

While running shoes are a good idea for a walker, they are a must for a jogger. The average runner (we use the words *runner* and *jogger* interchangeably) hits the ground with each foot about 800 times per mile. Each time you come down, you thrust your entire body weight onto your foot. Your ankles, knees, and hips must absorb the shock. Today's running shoes are designed to cushion the shock and prevent leg and foot injuries. They are also very comfortable. If you've never worn a pair of running shoes, you'll be pleasantly surprised when you try on your first pair and see just how springy and comfortable they are.

The shoe is by far the most important piece of equipment you need for running. In warm weather, you only need shorts and a T-shirt, preferably made of natural fibers to insure proper ventilation. Another layer of heavy cotton sweat pants and sweat shirt or warm-up jacket is a good idea for running in cooler weather. Put on gloves and a wool cap when the temperature drops below 35 or 40. Women should always wear brassieres; there are many types of special sports bras on the market today.

You'll find that you need less clothing than you might think when you run in cold weather. Once you get going, your body creates its own mini-environment. Even at temperatures below 30 degrees, you'll find yourself perspiring after you've run 10–15 minutes. You won't need more than a heavy sweat shirt and sweat pants, gloves, and a cap while running in all but the bitterest cold to keep warm. If the temperature is in the teens and the wind is blowing, the best thing to do is not run. The same holds true when temperatures are in the upper 90s with high humidity and air pollution. The idea is to remain healthy, not to risk more health problems by running in extremes of temperature.

The objectives in aerobic running are the same as in all other aerobic routines. You want to get yourself to the point where your heart is beating in your target zone for at least 20 minutes at a time 3 times per week. You need to stretch out, especially the leg muscles, for 5–10 minutes before running. Again, doing 6–8 sun salutations is a good way to get an overall stretch, as are the leg stretches described on p. 79.

As with the other aerobic routines, you should go very slowly for the first 5 minutes of running to give your muscles time to warm up. And you should greatly reduce your intensity for the last 5 minutes of running in order to help the muscles cool down. After you've finished running, don't just go about your business. Stretch out the leg muscles for at least 5 more minutes. Then you'll feel refreshed and relaxed and chances are, your muscles won't ache or stiffen up later.

Here are some other things to keep in mind if you're about to begin a running routine. As with walking, you should be running at a pace where you can carry on a conversation easily with someone alongside you. If you're panting heavily you are exerting yourself too much and chances are you're exceeding your target zone. Slow down. When you finish running, you should not be panting either, or out of breath. If you are, you're pushing yourself too hard. So the next time you run, cut back on your intensity.

Don't grit your teeth while you're running. Don't grimace.

Remember, you're out there to get away from the clenched-jawed pressures of your daily life that bring stress. The last thing you want to do is take part in an exercise that contributes more stress. Gritting your teeth is a sure sign that you're overdoing it. If you find yourself grimacing while you're running, just cut back on your pace and purposefully relax your facial muscles. It wouldn't hurt to smile a bit either.

Here's a good way to get started on an aerobics running regime. The first time out, don't even run at all. Just walk fairly briskly for about 15 minutes without stopping. See how you feel. Two days later, try walking for 10 minutes and then jogging very slowly for 5. Forget about reaching the target zone for now. Just concentrate on how you feel as you're running. Again, on your third time out during the first week, walk for 10 minutes and then run slowly for 5.

For the 3 sessions in your second week, walk for 5 minutes and try jogging for 10. If you feel very winded, go back to the 10-minute walk and 5-minute jogging routine. The third week, try jogging for 15 minutes straight. It doesn't matter how slowly you go, or how far you go, so long as you run steadily without stopping. Begin taking your pulse during the third week to see how you stand vis-à-vis your target zone. Be careful, and don't creep into the danger zone. If you do so, cut back on your intensity immediately.

By the fourth week, you should be trying to reach your target zone, and be running for 15–20 minutes without stopping. If you find this extremely taxing, try running for 15 minutes and walking briskly for 5. The next week, keep to the same schedule. Remember not to take any longer than two days between running sessions. A good running schedule might be Monday, Wednesday, and Friday, or Tuesday, Thursday, and Saturday. If you have the time to spare, the best schedule of all is to run 5 days a week while resting on weekends.

By the sixth week, you should be able to run for 20 minutes without stopping. If you keep up this regimen, in a few more weeks, you'll be able to run without undue discomfort for those 20 minutes. Don't get overanxious and run longer than 30 minutes at a time. Remember, you're still building up the strength in your legs. If you run too far before your leg muscles get developed, you risk permanently damaging your legs.

Keep taking your pulse regularly until you feel you know when you're in the target zone instinctively. Be alert for warnings from your body, and heed them. You'll soon find that running can be a relaxing way to get cardiovascular benefits while also giving yourself a secure, peaceful psychological feeling.

Cycling

Another aerobic routine that will help you combat stress is cycling—either on an indoor, stationary bicycle or on an outdoor rolling bike. The basic rules of aerobics apply to cycling. You need to get your heart into the target zone for at least 20 consecutive minutes at least 3 times per week. You should do at least 5 minutes of stretching exercises emphasizing the legs before you get on the bike, and another 5 minutes of stretching after you finish pedaling. For the first few minutes on the cycle, you should pedal easily, using this time as a warm-up. Then, after you've warmed up, you should pedal steadily for at least 20 minutes before cooling down with 5 final easy minutes on the bike.

Whether you choose an indoor stationary cycle or an outdoor rolling one is entirely up to you. Here are some things to keep in mind to help you make the choice. It can be difficult to plot out an aerobics course outdoors. You need to be pedaling continuously and steadily, but if you have hills, you'll be forced to pedal vigorously, spending extra effort trying to climb them. As you go down hills, you won't be expending any energy at all if you coast. An indoor cycle presents no such problems, and when you pedal indoors, there is no danger of being hit by cars or trucks. Moreover, you won't be at the mercy of the elements, as are outdoor cyclists who must endure wind, rain, and snow.

The basic drawback with indoor cycling is that it can be exceedingly boring. Outside bike riders can pedal through serene parks and on back roads and can therefore take in scenery while exercising. But indoor cyclists sit in the same spot for about half an hour at a stretch. There are some ways to enliven indoor-cycling routines. You can place your stationary bike in front of the TV set, for one thing. If you're cycling in the morning, you can catch the morning news on the tube and exercise at the same time. Or you can get an audio cassette machine with lightweight headphones and listen to your favorite music as you pedal. You can also prop a book, magazine, or newspaper on the handlebars and read while you cycle.

The only special equipment you need for cycling, of course, is either a sturdy indoor bike or a well-built 5-, 10-, or 12-speed outdoor one. You can buy special bicycling shoes, shocks, shorts, shirts, gloves, and helmets. None are necessary, although it is a good idea to wear a protective helmet when cycling outdoors. Don't wear running shoes with waffle soles because they can catch on the pedals and make you fall. As far as the rest of your cycling clothing is concerned, you can wear any type of lightweight, close-fitting, natural fiber clothing—a T-shirt and shorts will do.

It's important that when you buy a bike, you have it adjusted to fit your body. When you purchase a rolling bike, make sure that the salesperson adjusts the seat so that when your leg is fully extended with your toe on the pedal, there is a very slight bend in the knee. If the seat is adjusted too high or too low, you run the risk of injuring your knees. The seat also should be adjusted horizontally so that the handlebars are at arm's length from the seat. This will enable you to ride in a comfortable position that puts no strain on your upper body. When you buy an indoor cycle, there are two basic things to look for: Make sure that it is solid and sturdy, and that there is some sort of tension bar to adjust pedal pressure.

Swimming

There are several unique benefits of aerobic swimming. First and most important, swimming is one of the few aerobic routines that requires you to use your upper body muscles as well as your leg muscles. Also, swimming is a nonweight-bearing exercise. This means that since water holds you up, you don't have to put pressure on your legs as you do in walking, cycling, running, and dancing. That is why swimming is especially recommended for those with any sort of leg injury and for older persons.

Swimming, of course, provides the same cardiovascular benefits as do other aerobic exercises, and you go about your swimming program the same way you do the other aerobics: 5 minutes of stretching before you hop in the pool, 5 minutes of easy swimming to warm up, 20 minutes of target-zone swimming, 5 minutes of cooling down in the water and finally, a few minutes of out-of-the-water stretching.

The stretches should take in all the major muscle groups— arms, shoulders, back, chest, abdomen, and legs. As with the other aerobic routines, beginners should take it very slowly the first few weeks. Don't even try to get 20 straight minutes of swimming in. Just go as far as you can comfortably. Then rest. If you keep at your swimming regularly, you'll soon be able to swim easily for the required amount of time needed to get aerobic benefits.

Swimming does require you to get out of your house and make a trip to a health club, YMCA, or other facility. But swimming requires very little in the way of special equipment. A bathing suit is really all you'll need. Some pools require caps for those with long hair. If you have sensitive eyes, you may want to use special swimmers' goggles.

The experts say that aerobic swimmers should pick one stroke and stay with it. Most beginners find that the least demanding swimming stroke, the overhand crawl, is best. Don't experiment with other strokes until you've gotten your cardiovascular capacity to a high level and you want a change in your swimming routine.

Swimming can be very relaxing and enjoyable. Many regular swimmers find to their pleasant surprise that swimming gives them more than just cardiovascular benefits and muscle toning. They find that swimming helps them wash away the stressors of life and provides a general feeling of well-being.

Rope Skipping

The final aerobic routine we recommend, rope skipping, is not for everyone. It's very, very strenuous, and can be quite repetitive and monotonous. But it is also a very effective cardiovascular conditioner, and those in good physical shape may want to give it a try. But be warned: Rope skipping is very taxing, takes a great deal of effort, and will simply wear you out if you aren't in good shape to begin with. If you want to try rope skipping, follow the general aerobic rules: Stretch out for 5 minutes, start slowly, aim for 20 minutes in the target zone, finish with 5 minutes of cooling down, and another 5 minutes of stretching.

Strength Building

Thus far, we've covered two of the three basic components of a well-rounded exercise program: stretching and aerobics. The third part, strength-building exercises, is not as crucial as the others for fighting stress. But an exercise program is really not complete without at least some strength building—say a minimum of 10–15 minutes per week.

You should do some strength-building exercises because stronger muscles will help you in aerobics. Strong leg muscles, for example, will enable you to run, walk, dance, cycle, and swim longer and without undue fatigue. Strong muscles also reduce the possibility of injury. And a strong, well-conditioned body can give you a confident outlook on life based on the knowledge that you have strength and can take care of yourself if you need to call on your muscles in an emergency.

There are two basic types of strength-building exercises: isometric and isotonic. We do not recommend isometrics because each isometric exercise (in which you push or pull with all of your strength for a few seconds at a time) concentrates only on one or two muscles. You'd need to do at least a dozen different isometric exercises even to approach getting all-around muscle strength.

Lifting weights works to build strength in a few specific muscles. Therefore, a weight-training regime with free weights or with machines such as the Universal or Nautilus types, takes time—from 45 minutes to 90 minutes for a well-rounded session. You need to do 2 or 3 weight-training sessions a week to get any benefit. If you feel the desire to lift weights, the best thing to do is to sign up for a beginner's weight-training course at a gym. Learn the basics and then find a place where you can work out at the time of your choice with a program you've developed for yourself.

Calisthenics, which provide strength to the major muscle groups, can be integrated into your aerobic exercise programs easily. Calisthenics have one great advantage over isometrics and weight training for those trying to combat stress. Calisthenics are low-level exercises and therefore put very little stress on the cardiovascular system. When you lift weights or do isometrics, you greatly increase the demands on your heart—your blood pressure rises dramatically and your heart beat quickens. This is true also with calisthenics, but to a much lesser degree.

If you want to add calisthenics to your aerobics routine, try doing some sit-ups, push-ups, and pull-ups (if a bar is available) after you've cooled down. As with other forms of exercise, take it easy at first and work your way slowly up to about 30 sit-ups, 30-push-ups, and 10 pull-ups for each session.

1. Jim Fixx, *The Complete Book of Running* (New York: Random House, Inc., 1977), pp. 23–24.

10 / Diet, Nutrition, Obesity, Weight Control, and Stress

Nutrition can be a factor in stress management. It does appear that optimum levels of vitamins, minerals, carbohydrates, liquids (fats), proteins, and fiber are necessary in order to cope adequately with stressors.

Donald R. Morse and M. Lawrence Furst, *Stress for Success: A Holistic Approach to Stress and Its Management.*

Stress and diet have a dual relationship. On one hand, chronic stress can—and often does—influence the way we eat. On the other hand, how and what we eat can contribute to mental and physical stress.

Some of us, when faced with chronic stress, undereat. This can be physically harmful because stressful periods put extra demands on the body. During these times, you need a steady supply of nutrients to give your body energy to function smoothly. If you are under chronic stress for long periods of time, and you respond by undereating, you can significantly weaken your bodily defenses. This leaves you vulnerable to many types of disease.

Other people react to stress by overeating. This, too, can be harmful physically, especially when the overeating leads to obesity. According to Dr. Selye, obesity in certain persons may be a "manifestation of stress, especially in people with certain types of frustrating mental experiences. A person who does not get enough satisfaction from work or from his relations with other people may be driven to find consolation in almost anything that may provide comfort ...some people are driven to food just as others are driven to drink."[1]

It's easy to see how stress can cause us to over- or undereat. The problem is that being extremely thin or fat is definitely out of fashion in our society. Thus, the underweight or obese person is cast as an outsider, someone who does not fit in. This, in turn, can affect interpersonal relationships and have a broad bearing on how an individual feels about himself.

Obesity, which usually is defined as the bodily state in which you exceed your ideal weight by 20 percent or more, creates particularly serious physical problems. The obese person's excess poundage puts a strain on all the body's systems, especially the cardiovascular system. Obesity is universally recognized as one of the risk factors associated with heart disease.

How to Lose Weight

If you are overweight or obese, you should think seriously about trying to lose weight. Not only will losing weight be more healthful, but it could take away some of the psychological pressure inherent in being overweight in a society that glamorizes the slim-and-trim look.

The best way to lose weight, and to keep it off permanently, is to combine a regular exercise routine with a diet that is low in calories, fat, sodium, and processed foods, and high in whole grains and fresh fruits and vegetables. You won't lose weight overnight with this regime. But if you stick with it you will be rewarded. After a few months of exercising and watching your diet, you should see results.

Fad diets—the drinking man's diet, the Hollywood stars' diet, the whatever diet—do not work. In nearly all fad diets, you lose weight quickly—5 pounds in the first few days or 10 pounds the first week. But this is merely water loss. Once you stop the fad diet and return to your normal eating habits, you also return to your former weight.

There is a basic disagreement in medical circles today over how and why we lose weight. Many doctors believe that weight loss is a matter of simple mathematics: If you consume more calories than you burn up, you gain weight; if you burn up more calories than you consume, you lose weight.

The calorie-burning theory has been challenged by Dr. William Bennett, associate editor of the *Harvard Medical School Health Letter,* and Joel Gurin, managing editor of *American Health* magazine. In their 1982 book, *The Dieter's Dilemma: Eating Less and Weighing More,* Bennett and Gurin propound the "setpoint" theory of weight control. This holds that, in essence, each of us has a biological setpoint we are born with that controls our body weight because it "sets" the amount of fat in our cells, and that no amount of dieting can alter the setpoint.

For evidence, they point to several controlled studies. In one, prisoners were put on a diet extremely high in calories and fat, and were not permitted to exericse. The prisoners all gained a lot of weight. But once they were taken off the diet and allowed to eat as they chose, nearly all of them returned to the weight they started out with before the enforced high-calorie diet began. A similar result was found with a group put on a strict low-calorie diet combined with a regular exercise program. All the prisoners lost weight, but when they were allowed to eat and exercise any way they chose, nearly all of the prisoners' weight levels returned to just about where they were before the enforced dietary regime.

You probably know people who are very thin yet eat large amounts of food and never seem to gain weight. And you may know others who are overweight but eat very little. This is further evidence of the setpoint theory.

Bennett and Gurin claim that the only way to lower the setpoint is by engaging in regular exercise, especially the aerobic programs outlined in chapter 9. What happens when a person sticks with an aerobics program for a long period of time is that the body "sets" itself to be thinner. In this respect, the setpoint theory agrees with the calorie-counting theory of weight loss which also emphasizes exercise as a way to burn off calories.

The low-calorie, low-fat diet combined with exercise also provides another benefit. If you stick with this regime for several months, chances are it will bring about a series of changes in your life-style—a series of changes that should help you cope with stress, both mental and physical. If you are a smoker, for example, you should find that it is very hard to maintain your cigarette habit, exercise, and eat a healthy diet at the same time. Most smokers who undertake a diet-exercise regime soon give up smoking cigarettes.

The same thing is true with respect to excessive drinking and "recreational" drug abuse. These modes of behavior are simply not compatible with exercising. Most of those who take the step toward regular exercise and a healthy diet also jettison their alcohol or drug habits.

Here are some hints to help you begin a low-calorie, low-fat, healthful diet.

Salt

Whether you are overweight or underweight, obese, or at your ideal weight, you should be aware of how much salt you consume every day. The average American ingests from 2 to 5 teaspoons of salt per day. Forty percent of that salt is sodium—a substance which increases the body's total volume of blood and raises blood pressure. High blood pressure (hypertension) is one of the risk factors in heart disease.

About 60 million Americans have some form of high blood pressure. It is the main cause of the 500,000 cases of strokes and 170,000 stroke deaths that take place in this country every year. And high blood pressure probably is a factor in many of the 1,250,000 heart attacks suffered by Americans each year, and the 550,000 heart attack deaths which take place annually.

The body needs some sodium to maintain blood pressure and volume and to control water passage through the body. If we don't get enough sodium in extremely hot weather, we risk heat exhaustion, cramps, and in some extreme cases, death from heat prostration. But just how much sodium do we need? The amount varies from person to person, depending primarily on body weight. The average adult needs only about 200 milligrams of sodium a day—the amount contained in one tenth of a teaspoon of salt. This is an amount most of us get from sodium found naturally in food and water. If you are like most Americans and consume 2 teaspoons of salt every day, you are ingesting about 24 times the amount of sodium your body needs.

If you want to reduce your sodium intake, you should look at the food you eat every day. Nutritionists claim that only about a third of the sodium we consume is added to food at the table, so using less salt at mealtime won't do much to make a dramatic difference in our salt consumption. Nearly half of our sodium intake comes from processed foods such as canned or dried soups, canned vegetables, pickles, olives, and frozen dinners. And, as some people are shocked to discover, cake and bread also contain moderate to heavy doses of sodium.

The best way to get your salt consumption down to a healthy level of about 8,000 milligrams a day (those with high blood pressure should consume less than 2,000 milligrams a day) is to avoid eating high-sodium processed foods. Better yet, eliminate all processed food from your diet in favor of fresh foods. Fresh lima beans, for example, contain only 2 milligrams of sodium per cup, while canned limas have 450 milligrams of sodium per cup.

You can easily find low-sodium or sodium-free products in most grocery stores or in health food stores. Or you can buy salt substitutes. But these substances should be avoided because they tend to have heavy amounts of potassium and other artificial additives.

Probably the best way to avoid excessive sodium consumption is to use whole foods (fresh fruits, vegetables, grains, legumes, and nuts), never add salt when cooking, sprinkle it only lightly on food at the table, and experiment with combinations of herbs and spices, and lemon and lime juice as flavorings.

Fat in the Diet

Another villain in today's typical American diet is fat. As is the case with sodium, the body needs some fat in order to exist. Fats are used to transport fat-soluble vitamins throughout the body. Fat also serves as a cushioning agent for the internal organs. But, as also is the case with sodium, most of us eat too much fat each day. Excessive fat buildup in the body can be very dangerous to your health.

The average American consumes about 105 grams of fat per day—about twice as much as the body needs. These fats are of two basic kinds: saturated and unsaturated. Animal fats—those which contain cholesterol—are saturated. The foods with the highest concentrations of saturated fat are beef, pork, lamb, bacon, ham, milk, cheese, butter, and eggs. There is less fat in turkey, chicken, and fish. Most vegetables, nuts, and grains contain unsaturated fat.

It has yet to be proven scientifically that unsaturated fats are better for you than saturated fats. But most nutritionists recommend that we cut down on our fat intake, especially fats that contain cholesterol, because of the link between excessive levels of certain types of cholesterol in the blood and heart disease.

The American Heart Association recommends that we ingest unsaturated fats whenever possible, and that we should not eat more than 3 egg yolks a week; use low or nonfat milk; and eat only lean meats, fish, and poultry.

Sugar

Sugar, too, is a substance (chemically called sucrose) that our bodies need. Sucrose is an energy source. But we Americans have a very sweet tooth. The average American consumes more than 125 pounds of sugar a year, most of which is highly refined. The consequences of ingesting this large amount of refined sugar (commonly contained in "empty calorie," or junk foods) include physical ailments such as tooth decay, obesity, diabetes, and hypoglycemia.

The best way to cut down on sugar is to stop adding refined sugar to foods and drinks at the table. Some of us are so used to sprinkling sugar on our morning cereal or grapefruit, or in our coffee or tea that we have no idea what these foods taste like without the added sugar. Just as an experiment, the next time you reach for the sugar bowl, try to remember what the food you are about to eat tasted like without sugar. If you can't remember, try eating the food with only a tiny bit of sugar or with none at all. This is one way not only to rediscover the taste of your food, but to wean yourself off of heavy sugar consumption.

Colas and other soft drinks contain large amounts of sugar. One way to cut back on your sugar intake is to cut out all soft drinks. Here's one method you may want to try. Make a vow to do without drinking any type of soft drink for a month. Try substituting fruit juice (the all-natural kind only, not the fruit drinks with added sugar), club soda, skimmed milk or mineral water when the soft drink urge hits. If you avoid soft drinks for a month, it's a good bet that when you taste one again you'll discover just how oversweetened it is. The overwhelming sweet taste just might cause you to give up soft drinks on the spot.

Giving up refined sugar and honey (which is mostly sugar) doesn't mean you have to give up sweet foods. If you eliminate processed sugar from your diet, you'll gain a new appreciation for the natural sweetness of oranges, bananas, pineapples, mangoes, papayas, and other fruits, melons, and even sweet vegetables such as tomatoes, sweet peppers, and sweet potatoes.

Caffeine

Yet another potentially unhealthy substance many of us ingest in large quantities is caffeine. But caffeine—unlike sodium, sucrose, and fat—is something the human body has no biological need for. Caffeine is a chemical stimulant that is found naturally in coffee beans, tea leaves, coca beans, and kola nuts. It is added to over-the-counter and prescription drugs, most often painkillers and stimulants. It also is added to cola drinks and to other soft drinks.

Caffeine stimulates the central nervous system, causing the heart and lungs to quicken their normal paces. It also clears the mind and combats fatigue.

Medical science does not know for sure the long-term consequences of excessive caffeine intake. But the drug has been implicated in a number of health problems, including birth defects, bladder cancer, breast disorders in women, and hyperactivity in children. In 1980, the U.S. Food and Drug Administration officially warned pregnant women to "avoid caffeine-containing foods and drugs, or to use them sparingly" because of the possibility that excessive caffeine consumption may cause birth defects.

It's easy to spot the high caffeine areas in our diets. But it is not always easy to cut them out. Heavy caffeine users can experience caffeine withdrawal, featuring headaches, nausea, and other symptoms, if they try to quit cold turkey. The best way to cut out caffeine is to do it gradually but purposefully. Try setting up a schedule with goals on a weekly basis. You can also try switching over to decaffeinated beverages or herbal teas.

Food Additives

A word on food additives. Nearly all food additives, especially artificial colors and artificial flavors, have no nutritive value. They are used in processed foods to keep them on the shelves longer or to dress up their taste or appearance. They, in short, are not there for consumers, but for food manufacturers. It's best to stay away from all foods that have artificial ingredients, and leave it at that.

What to Eat

Now that we've gone over what *not* to eat, the question remains: "What should we eat?" We've all heard it a thousand times, but it's true nevertheless: We should try to eat a balanced diet every day, consisting of fruits, vegetables, dairy products, grains, nuts, cereals, and seeds. The diet should be balanced with proteins, carbohydrates, fats and fiber.

The best sources of protein are those foods containing low amounts of fat such as fish, poultry, legumes, and low-fat yogurt and cheeses, such as cottage cheese. We should get most of our carbohydrates from vegetables, fruits, whole grain flour, and cereal grains, and our fat from unsaturated vegetable oils.

Here are some hints on how to replace processed foods with natural ones to ensure that your diet contains all the nutrients contained in whole foods without any of the excessive salt, sugar, fat, or artificial additives of over-processed foods.

Use whole grains rather than refined flour or cereal. In place of all-purpose flour, try whole wheat pastry flour or other whole grain flours such as rye flour. In place of processed, sugar-laden breakfast cereals, substitute cereals made without sugar, such as shredded wheat or rolled oats.

Use honey, pure maple syrup, unsulfured molasses, or fruit juices and purees in place of refined sugar. Try combinations of herbs, lemon juice, or garlic, in place of salt. Use vegetable oils instead of animal fat in cooking. Try to incorporate more raw foods into your diet, especially uncooked fruits and vegetables. Give seeds, sprouts, wheat germ, and brewer's yeast a place in your diet. Avoid whole milk products, including whole milk cheeses. Substitute low-fat milk, low-fat yogurt, or low-fat or goat cheeses for whole milk cheeses. Avoid red meat in favor of turkey, chicken, and fish. Avoid highly processed meats.

Your diet should not be filled with overcooked foods. Steam vegetables instead of boiling them. This seals in the vitamins and minerals rather than boiling them away. The flavors will be tastier and even the colors brighter when you steam (or very lightly sauté) vegetables. Avoid deep-fried foods. Baked potatoes are preferable to fried potatoes; poached eggs are better than fried eggs.

Give vegetarian meals a chance. Try going one day a week without eating meat or fish. Your vegetarian day might include whole grain cereal with low-fat milk and fruit for breakfast. Lunch could be a peanut butter and honey sandwich on whole wheat bread with a piece of fruit for dessert. For dinner, you could have a fresh garden salad with oil and vinegar dressing and a pasta dish with cheese or tomato sauce or a legume-based dish such as vegetarian chili, bean tacos, or lentil stew. For a snack, try raw almonds and raisins or popcorn with only a little bit of salt.

You may find that you enjoy the nonmeat diet. If you want to continue it, check out one or two of the scores of vegetarian cookbooks available today. Most include sections on how to eat a completely balanced diet without meat. One way to be sure you get enough B vitamins in a vegetarian diet is to take brewer's yeast, either in powder form mixed into food or in tablet form. Vegetarians who eat milk, eggs, butter, and cheese usually receive all the vitamins and minerals they need. You can also supplement a basic vegetarian diet with a small amount of fish or chicken if you feel you need an extra protein boost.

One of the best meat substitutes and one which contains hardly any fat but is very high in protein is tofu—a fermented soybean cake found in all Oriental grocery stores and in an increasing number of regular grocery stores. Tofu is inexpensive and can be prepared in dozens of different ways. It has been a dietary staple in Japan and China for centuries. An easy way to prepare tofu is to cut it into bite-size pieces and gently sauté them in butter or sunflower oil with bits of ginger, garlic, and sesame seeds. Then serve the tofu with steamed vegetables over brown rice.

If you follow the low-fat, low-sodium, low-sugar natural foods diet you'll be in for plenty of benefits: You should feel light and strong, not overstuffed. And you will prepare your body to do its best to fight off stress.

---

1. Selye; *Stress of Life*, p. 265.

11 / Breathing and Relaxation

> Emotional states and breathing patterns are very much interrelated...slow, rhythmic breathing can turn an anxious mental state into one of relative tranquility and release the body from many of the other adverse effects of anxiety.
>
> Kenneth R. Pelletier, *Mind as Healer, Mind as Slaver.*

As we have seen, deep breathing is an integral part of the stress reduction techniques of yoga, meditation, stretching, and relaxation exercises. But, as we will now see, breathing in and of itself also can be a relaxing antidote to stress.

Slow, rhythmic, abdominal breathing, as Dr. Pelletier states, is one key to fighting stress. This chapter presents several breathing exercises—ones you can use as daily relaxation regimes or intermittently on those occasions in everyday life when you need to relax.

As we saw in previous chapters, deep diaphragmatic breathing involves not just the lungs, chest, and throat, but also the abdominal region. This is a type of breathing most of us do *not* do. In order to breathe diaphragmatically, we, in essence, have to relearn how to breathe. Luckily, it is not difficult to learn how to breathe diaphragmatically, and nearly everyone can pick it up soon after learning the basics.

Here's a good way to learn. Put your right hand palm down on the upper part of your chest, just below your throat. Place the left palm directly in the middle of your stomach. Now, with your mouth closed, exhale deeply. You should feel your left hand move in as your stomach deflates. If you don't feel this, and if your chest is moving first, you are not breathing correctly.

Now take a deep inhalation. Your left hand should move out as your stomach expands like a balloon. This is a good way to practice deep diaphragmatic breathing, keeping your hands in these positions, breathing in and out, and making sure you have very little movement in the chest and that the focus of the breath is in the abdomen.

In hatha yoga, the most common deep-breathing exercise is called pranayama. *Prana* is the Sanskrit word for "life," and the yogic deep-breathing exercises facilitate the infusion of fresh life into the system. How? Well, each deep breath brings with it a large infusion of fresh air. If you learn how to do the deep breathing correctly, you can actually increase the amount of fresh air taken into your body sevenfold compared to normal breathing. This new air helps bring large amounts of life-giving oxygen to each organ of the body.

Conversely, the deep breathing rapidly eliminates large quantities of stale air. The deep breathing, in effect, acts as a supercharger to the body, as it eliminates spent fuel to boost performance.

At the same time, deep breathing is a relaxation exercise. It helps mitigate stress the same way the other relaxation regimes do: by slowing down the bodily functions such as the heartbeat, blood pressure, and so on that tend to get sped up when we're under stress. In addition, deep breathing calms the mind, giving it a refreshing change of pace from the stressful world we live in.

You may use deep-breathing techniques any time during the day when you feel the need to get your act together, and to slow down and get a hold of yourself. The next time you watch a baseball game, you'll notice that many players take deep breaths just before they hit or pitch. And basketball players often take a deep breath or two before shooting a foul shot. These players have learned that deep breathing can get the body ready to perform, and relax them before a big moment.

You may not be called on to hit an important foul shot in the big game, but chances are, you will find the need to calm yourself down—maybe just before a meeting with the boss, before delivering a speech, waiting in the dentist's office, or even getting ready to cook a big dinner for the in-laws.

To use deep breathing to calm yourself in these and other potentially stressful situations, simply walk away from the action for a few minutes to be alone. Sit in a chair (or stand if you have no choice), close your eyes, calm yourself, and then expel all the stale air out of your body in one deep, smooth, slow exhalation. Hold your body still for a second while the air is out, and then gently but firmly inhale a large dose of fresh air. You'll actually be able to feel a cool, clean sensation in your lungs as you inhale fresh, clean air. Take 2 or 3 of these deep breaths anytime you feel the need to. They're sure to help you relieve tension.

Before we get to the regular, daily deep-breathing exercises, there are a few general things to keep in mind. The best position for deep breathing is either in a comfortable cross-legged seated position on the floor, in a comfortable chair, or lying on your back on the floor. Yoga teachers say that the best way to do breathing exercises is the cross-legged position, but lying down or sitting in a chair will suffice for the simple, relaxing breathing programs we advocate.

Five to 10 minutes of these breathing exercises are all you need for each daily session. Beginners should attempt to do only 2 or 3 minutes at first. As is the case with any new routine, you should begin slowly and only gradually take on more. Remember not to overstrain. There is less of a chance that you'll do yourself bodily harm with these exercises than with any of the other relaxing exercises in this book. But don't forget that the breathing exercises work with delicate organs: the lungs, the heart, and the nerves. So it's wise to take it especially easy at first.

You want to wear light, loose clothing for the breathing exercises. If you are at work, just loosen your garments if they fit tightly, especially around the midsection. Do the exercises in a quiet place, where you'll have no interruptions. Keep the lights dim, don't play any music, and try to keep your mind only on what you are doing at all times. Don't let your mind wander.

Simple Deep-Breathing Exercises

The first exercise is the basic, simple, deep, relaxing breathing exercise. You already know the basics. And that's about all you have to do. Close your eyes and keep them shut. While sitting or lying down, make sure you're completely relaxed. Now exhale slowly to the count of 5. Count to yourself: "1, 1,000, 2, 1,000," and so on. As soon as you've exhaled completely, inhale slowly to another 5 counts. Exaggerate the abdominal inhalation. Feel your stomach expand. Then exhale again, feeling your collarbone drop a tiny bit, your chest contract ever so slightly, and then your stomach draw in.

Keep your breath moving in one continuous flow, counting

5 long seconds for each inhalation and for each exhalation. Your inhalations should begin from the abdomen; the exhalations from the top of the lungs. Try this routine for a few minutes each day. Then after a week or so, expand to 5 rounds. When you feel comfortable, try 10 minutes of the concentrated deep breathing. After you finish, sit still for another minute or two. Feel your breathing return to normal. Then, before rising, take one more nice deep abdominal breath, and get up and go on with the business of the day.

Alternative Nostril Breathing

This is a type of breathing exercise practiced in hatha yoga. Yogis claim that alternative nostril breathing helps keep the mind alert and aids digestion and sleep. This may or may not be true. But alternative nostril breathing has helped many persons get relief from tension headaches. And, if nothing else, you can use these exercises as a change of pace from the simple deep-breathing regime just described.

It's best to do alternative nostril breathing while sitting, rather than lying down. Begin by taking a few deep abdominal breaths. Then let your breath return to normal, and with your left hand in your lap, place the thumb of your right hand on your nose to close off the right nostril. Exhale slowly through the left nostril to the count of 8. After that exhalation, keep the thumb over the right nostril and inhale deeply to a count of 4 through the left nostril. When you hit 4 seconds, close off the left nostril with the pinkie and ring finger of your right hand. Keep the middle two fingers tucked into the palm. Keep the right thumb on the right nostril.

Hold your breath with both nostrils closed off for 16 seconds. Then, keeping the left nostril closed off with the same two fingers, release the thumb from the right nostril and exhale to a count of 8. Then inhale through the right nostril to a count of 4, and close off the right nostril with the thumb as you hold the breath again for 16 seconds. Next, exhale to a count of 8 through the left nostril. When you inhale again for 4 seconds through the left nostril, you have completed one round of alternate nostril breaths.

Beginners should do 3 or 4 rounds at first. Later, after a few weeks' practice, you can move up to 6 or 8 rounds. The aim is to do 10–12 rounds a day. If you have trouble holding the inhalations, exhalations, or the in-between breaths, try lowering them to 2 seconds for the inhalation, 4 seconds for the exhalations, and 8 seconds holding the breath between rounds. If you're extraordinarily comfortable with the 4–8–16 second formula, move up to 5 seconds for inhalations, 10 seconds for exhalations, and 20 seconds for holding your breath.

You can do the alternative nostril breaths by themselves or integrate them into a yoga routine, either before you start the postures or after you've finished. In some yoga routines, the alternative nostril breaths are followed by a rapid, bellow-type breathing technique. This type of deep breathing is said to provide many benefits, but can cause some persons to hyperventilate and pass out. If you try the rapid breathing and feel even slightly dizzy or nauseous, stop immediately.

Rapid Deep Breathing

You do the rapid deep breathing in a seated position. Sitting up straight with your eyes closed, hands in your lap, begin inhaling and exhaling deeply and slowly. On your third or fourth exhalation, expel the air with a quick, sharp breath. This sharp breath should emanate from your stomach. As soon as you exhale forcefully, take a quick, short inhalation. This inhalation should come naturally; it won't require much exertion or movement. Concentrate therefore on the forceful exhalations. Count 30 rapid breaths. Then slow down the breathing and push all the breath out of your stomach in one long, deep exhalation. Hold your breath for a few seconds. Then inhale very deeply. Try holding your breath for 20 seconds. Then exhale fully. Take another deep inhalation and then let your breath return to normal. Try another round of the rapid deep breathing; this time, try to hold your breath for 30 seconds.

The object is to do 3 rounds, holding your breath for 30, 60, and then 90 seconds following each rapid round of breathing. You won't be able to reach this right away. Expect to practice the exercise daily for several weeks before you get your lungs built up to hold the breath for the 30, 60, and 90 seconds. If you can't get the hang of it right away, and still want to try to master the routine, take a yoga course where you can get personalized instruction.

12 / Stress and Sleep

> The stress of a day of hard work can make you
> sleep like a log or it can keep you awake all night.
>
> Dr. Hans Selye,
> *The Stress of Life.*

As Dr. Selye notes, stress and sleep are interconnected in both positive and negative ways. Too much of the wrong kind of stress during the day can lead to sleep problems, especially insomnia. But the right kind of stress, such as physical and/or mental effort that lead to a successful, satisfying conclusion, can prepare the body and mind for untroubled sleep.

Doctors think that at least a quarter of the adult population of America—perhaps as many as 50 million people—has problems with sleep. By far the most common sleeping problem is insomnia, either early onset onsomnia, in which you cannot fall asleep when you go to bed, or early-awakening insomnia when you wake up in the middle of the night and can't fall back asleep.

There are several other kinds of sleep problems. These do not involve being unable to sleep, but have to do with being unable to stay awake. Some persons are afflicted with a condition in which they fall asleep suddenly at odd times during the day. Others are bothered by the serious problem of being unable to breathe while sleeping.

Insomnia, the most common sleeping problem, has innumerable causes, both mental and physical. Some persons cannot sleep because of physical ailments such as arthritis or breathing disorders. But it appears as if the majority of insomnia sufferers cannot sleep well because of stress-related psychological and emotional problems.

Psychologists often find cases of persistent insomnia caused by an individual's temporary response to stress—either positive stress such as a wedding, or negative stress such as an impending divorce. At first, the stress causes the person to be too keyed up to sleep well. Then, the temporary sleeplessness caused by the stress feeds on itself, causing more and more sleepless nights. Once a bad sleeping pattern becomes a habit—say after three weeks or so—it becomes very, very difficult to overcome.

Another type of stress-related insomnia is an untreated case of depression or anxiety which boils over at night and causes sleeplessness. As we have seen, psychologists think that depression—and to a lesser extent anxiety—is caused when someone represses and bottles up emotions. Often the depressed or anxious person internalizes feelings during the day, but these emotions and worries come to the surface at night and bring insomnia. "Insomniac patients often have difficulty expressing and controlling their aggressive feelings," writes Dr. Anthony Kales, director of the Sleep Research and Treatment Center at the Pennsylvania State University Medical Center. "Going to sleep represents a loss of control, and insomnia is a defense against this fear."[1]

How to Relieve Stress that Causes Sleep Problems

There are a number of things you can do if you are among the tens of millions of Americans with stress-related sleep problems.

One particular problem, Dr. Selye claims, is overworking the body or mind to the point of exhaustion. This is because when we get keyed up—whether from exercising vigorously or from arguing vociferously—our bodies react by exhibiting the classic stress-induced physical changes, including the release of hormones designed to keep us operating at top mental and physical efficiency. So the keyed up mind and the tensed up muscles can make sleep difficult.

The answer, psychologists say, is to avoid tasks that are overly repetitive, especially after you are already tired. Don't take that report home from the office if you're exhausted at the end of a long workday. And don't do that stack of dirty dishes late at night after a hectic dinner party. "Remember that stress is the great equalizer of biologic activities and if you use the same parts of the body or mind over and over again, the only means nature has to force you out of the groove is general...stress," comments Dr. Selye.[2]

Insomnia itself is a stressor. This is a reason why insomnia builds up on itself. It produces emotional arousal at night, tiredness the following day, and then another bout of insomnia the next night—a vicious cycle that for many becomes worse the longer it manifests itself.

How Much Sleep Do We Need?

The old saying that we need 8 hours of sleep every night, medical opinion now holds, is true. There are many variables, including age, sex, and physical condition, in determining the optimal amount of sleep. But doctors have conducted studies indicating that those who get an average of 8 hours of sleep per night tend to have fewer psychological and physical problems than those who sleep 6 hours or less and those who sleep 9 hours or more.

It's also important to remember that the ideal amount of sleep is a highly individual thing. Younger persons tend to sleep longer than older persons. In addition, you need more than your normal amount of sleep during periods of stress, depression, or increased mental activity. The extra sleep during these times acts as a sort of curative for the problems that can be caused by being unable to cope with stressful events.

How to Get a Good Night's Sleep

The environment you create for yourself in your bedroom has a great deal to do with how you sleep. You want a well-ventilated room without too much noise, light, cold, or heat.

Aside from avoiding getting too keyed up late in the day, you should also avoid some other insomnia-enhancing things: alcohol, cigarettes, and coffee. Drinking alcohol provides a mental illusion of tiredness, but it is only a temporary condition. If you go to sleep drunk, you risk being jolted awake in the middle of the night after your body absorbs the alcohol. Doctors think that alcohol is a major contributor to insomnia; many alcoholics sleep only several hours a night.

The first thing some people do after failing to fall asleep is get out of bed and light up a cigarette. Getting out of bed might not be such a bad idea, but lighting up a cigarette is one of the worst things you can do. Not only is cigarette smoking in general harmful to your health, but the nicotine in tobacco is a stimulant. Medical studies, including the work of Dr. Kales at Penn State, have shown that smoking makes it harder to combat the effects of insomnia. Studies also show that smokers who had sleep problems reported dramatic improvement in sleeping after they gave up cigarettes.

It's pretty easy to see why drinking coffee or other caffeinated beverages works against sleeping. Caffeine is one of the most powerful stimulants you can ingest. Over-the-counter "stay awake" pills typically contain large dosages of the substance. Remember that most types of tea—except herbal teas—also contain caffeine, as do cola and other soft drinks (check the label), chocolate, and a number of over-the-counter and prescription drugs, primarily pain relievers and stimulants.

Something else to avoid if at all possible are sleeping pills, known as hypnotics. These substances should be taken only as a very last resort. The reason: You can easily become dependent on them to get you through the night. Moreover, hypnotics actually *cause* insomnia for some people because the drug's effects can wear off during the middle of the night, leaving the user wide-awake. Another thing. Sleeping pills when mixed with alcohol can be lethal. If you think you are dependent on sleeping pills and want to kick the habit, consult your physician. It can be very harmful just to stop taking the pills on your own.

The experts also say that exercise is a good antidote to insomnia—providing you exercise in the proper manner. This means not doing any stimulating exercise, such as aerobics, calisthenics, or weight training, three hours before bedtime. If you follow the balanced exercise regime recommended in chapter 6—and remember not to do the strenuous ones late at night—you may just enhance your ability to sleep soundly.

Other ways to fight off insomnia include going to bed *only* when you are sleepy and using the bed *only* for sleeping and sexual activity. Do not read, watch television, eat, or sit in bed and worry. These activities will only prolong insomnia. Don't go to bed when you're not sleepy. Wait as long as you can when you feel sleep coming on, and then go to bed. And don't take naps during the day if you have a problem with insomnia. This is a good way to upset your "biological clock" and prolong insomnia.

If you have trouble getting to sleep right away, the experts say you can try the tried-and-true method of counting sheep, or use the relaxation autosuggestion techniques described in chapter 6. Or use the yoga corpse pose, lying on your back with your arms out to your sides palms up, and your legs apart 12–18 inches. Just stay motionless and try meditating, although you should not couple your regular meditation practice with trying to sleep. These techniques induce sleep because they help you concentrate on relaxing, and get you away from dwelling on the stressors of life.

If you cannot fall asleep within 10–15 minutes of the time you go to bed, it's usually no use to stay in bed. Sleep specialists recommend that you get out of bed, get out of the bedroom, and get involved in some bland activity such as reading or watching television. But don't watch an exciting show. You can even fix a light snack—nothing heavy—but don't drink tea, coffee, or alcohol. Try warm milk or herbal tea. Whatever you do, don't do any office homework. After your light snack, you should soon begin to feel drowsy. If you do, wait a bit and then go back to bed.

If these methods fail, you might consider seeking professional counseling. Today, there are not only doctors who specialize in treating sleep disorders, but there are more than 100 sleep disorder centers across the country. Treatment at these centers usually is of the holistic variety. You are examined by a battery of specialists, from neurologists to psychiatrists. You are then given an individualized treatment that often includes psychotherapy or medication.

Other sleeping problems, including narcolepsy, excessive daytime sleeping, and sleep apnea, in which breathing actually stops during sleep, are much less common, but potentially much more dangerous than insomnia. If you suffer from these ailments, the best thing to do is consult a physician.

1. Anthony Kales, writing in the *American Handbook of Psychiatry*, ed. S. Arieti, vol. 7 (1981), p. 428.
2. Selye, *Stress of Life*, p. 424.

13 / Hints on How to Help You Cope with Everyday Stress

The previous chapters described five different programs—relaxation exercises, meditation, yoga, physical exercise, and deep breathing—that you can practice on a regular basis to combat stress. This chapter outlines some steps you can take to cope with stressful matters any time you want to. We also present a set of calming, stress-reducing activities you can use whenever you feel particularly hassled by stressful situations.

Water Treatment

The Japanese are big believers in bathing as a way both to cleanse the body and calm the mind. In this country you have the choice of half a dozen water-treatment methods to use when you're feeling overly frustrated and feel the desire to put the calming qualities of water to good use.

Just taking a hot bath can do wonders. A great escape from the outside world all of us can enjoy is filling a tub with hot water, adding some "bubble bath," lighting a candle, burning some incense, and just soaking in the water with perhaps some soothing music in the background. Take a glass of wine and sip it in the tub, or curl up with a novel. You'll be escaping your frustrations and worries and the warm water will help relax tense, stiff muscles.

Saunas, steam baths, whirlpools, hot tubs, and sensory deprivation tanks also work to relax the muscles. There is nothing like half an hour of sitting in a bubbling whirlpool after a physical workout to loosen stiff muscles and calm your thoughts. Saunas and steam baths provide a more rigorous water-heat relaxer. You sweat away your troubles either with the extremely dry heat of a sauna or with the wet heat of a steam bath. Doctors do warn that those with heart ailments should avoid saunas and steam baths. If you feel any discomfort while in a sauna or steam bath, you should leave immediately, drink some cool water, and stay away until you feel no dizziness, nausea, or other discomfort.

There is very little danger of physical problems from hot tubs and sensory deprivation tanks. The only problem with these two great tension easers is that they are very costly to install in your home and not many people can afford them. But there are hot tub emporiums where you can go and soak, either alone or with a friend or group of friends. Sensory deprivation tanks are womblike environments in which you enclose yourself while lying in the fetal position in a few inches of warm water. As you close your eyes and sink into the soundless, lightless environment, your body will receive all the relaxation benefits needed to combat stress. Inside the tank your bodily systems slowly calm down and both the body and mind relax thoroughly.

Massage

Anyone who has had a deep-muscle massage—or any other type of massage at the hands of a trained masseuse or masseur—does not have to be told how relaxing a good massage can be. In deep-muscle massage, the muscles, tendons, joints, skin, and fat tissues are manipulated to the point where they loosen up and all tension is dissipated. Those who are extremely sensitive might not be able to appreciate the benefits of certain types of deep-muscle massage because the manipulation sometimes causes more than a little pain.

Pets

Recent psychological studies have begun to uncover evidence that those who care for pets, especially dogs and cats, are better able to cope with the stressors of life. There are two basic reasons for this. First, taking responsibility for the care and feeding of an animal gets a person away from always being concerned with himself. Second, if you give love and attention to a pet, chances are, the pet will return the affection. Having an affectionate animal around who responds to you can be very calming and satisfying, especially when you are feeling lonesome. Your animal will always be there when you need attention and affection.

The physical act of stroking or petting a dog or cat can be therapeutic. It provides the animal with the intuitive knowledge that it is being cared for. It also gives you the calming feeling of warmth, affection, and interdependence with a reliable, trusting being.

Gardening

Just as taking care of pets can be rewarding, so too can tending another type of living organism—an outdoor vegetable or flower garden. Although time-consuming, it is not usually physically draining, and the rhythmical quality of working in the garden is especially helpful in mitigating the effects of stress.

And, then, of course, there is the ultimate reward, the fruits of your labor so to speak—the food you grow. Getting in touch with nature through nurturing a garden through the seasons certainly is a positive step anyone can take to get away from the tension-filled, pressure situations in life.

You can achieve the same results with a flower garden, by the way, or even working with indoor plants. Caring for flowers provides an aesthetic bonus when you see your work pay off in blooming colors and fragrances that calm the mind and soothe the senses.

Diversions

We've all heard the old expression, All work and no play makes you a dull person. And that adage makes sense. But many persons seem to ignore the advice; for them life is one long, continuous working day. It is necessary for all of us to figure out when we should work and when we should rest, loaf, play, or just take a break.

We mentioned in chapter 12 that those with insomnia should not take naps during the day. But it's perfectly OK for you to take naps if you don't have insomnia or other sleep problems, especially when you feel particularly tired or if you've missed your normal amount of sleep, say, on a weekend afternoon after you've stayed up late the night before and are planning another late night that evening. If you do take a nap, don't sleep any longer than 15 or 20 minutes, certainly not more than half an hour.

Aside from naps, it's a good idea to take regular breaks during your working day. If you feel yourself getting overwrought, tense, or otherwise frustrated, stop whatever you're doing and remove yourself from the action. Take a walk around the block if you have to. Go to another room. The important thing is to get away physically from the environment and the work that is causing your tension, if only for 5 minutes. This will give your system time to recuperate, relax, and refresh itself before you tackle the job again.

Leave room in your life for recreation. We're talking about getting involved in hobbies, going to the movies, watching television, reading, or visiting friends. As simple as this sounds, and as much common sense as it makes, there are those who neglect to take time to get away from their stressful situations. And they suffer for it.

Just getting interested in something other than work, family, and friends is enough. It can be a hobby such as antique collecting, following sports teams, or taking ballroom dancing lessons—anything that gets you totally out of your everyday pattern.

There is nothing wrong with just plain loafing every once in a while. Just lying around in a hammock staring at the sky, sitting on the front porch watching the world go by, taking a leisurely walk through the park, or sitting back in your easy chair with your eyes closed listening to music can give you a needed break from the anxiety-producing noises and worries of life.

Vacations

Don't neglect vacations. There is nothing better for "getting away from it all" than actually getting away—to another city, another part of the country, or even overseas. Your stressful life events will seem inconsequential and far removed when you leave your everyday surroundings.

Of course, there are some built-in stresses involved in vacations. There are reservations to make, planes to catch, and dozens of details to see to. But, if you go into a vacation or holiday with the attitude that you will have a relaxing time, you undoubtedly will have a relaxing time. Expect and plan for delays and frustrations. That way, you will be able to handle them with a minimal amount of frustration when they do occur. If you want to avoid unexpected and possibly unpleasant experiences, take your vacation somewhere you've been before, someplace where you're comfortable, where you know the routine, where there won't be unpleasant surprises, and where there will be very few anxious moments.

Letting it Out

Don't keep things bottled up. Talk out your troubles and problems with someone as often as possible. Talk things over with a close friend, a doctor, a religious counselor, or a member of your family. Or write down what's on your mind in a journal or diary. Talking or writing about your troubles often makes you realize how relatively insignificant and commonplace they are.

And remember it's all right to express your emotions. In fact, it can be quite harmful to keep your feelings internalized since they can turn into physical ailments and mental problems such as anxiety and depression. So express that anger—in an appropriate manner. Don't scream at your spouse, children, or co-workers. Channel your anger constructively by exercising vigorously (if you're in good shape), or by splitting wood, punching a punching bag, or beating a rug. Just taking a walk can sometimes allow you to vent steam.

Remember, too, that it's perfectly all right to cry. So often, our first reaction to overwhelmingly sad news is to stifle our tears. But when you feel tears coming on, let them fly; you'll notice how relieved you'll feel afterward.

Try doing something altruistic. It's a way of escaping from a wholly self-centered life-style—from always thinking about yourself. You can volunteer to work with the handicapped or mentally ill one night a week, or even to baby-sit for your neighbor's children. In fact, you'll find that helping others will actually help you get your mind off your problems.

14 / Professional Stress Counseling

> Psychotherapy certainly is not always needed to combat stress. But it often can be a valuable aid...it can be useful...for stress-provoked anxiety. It need not take the form of extended classic Freudian psychoanalysis, with years spent on the couch. The range of professional help for emotional problems is much broader now.
>
> Executive Health Examiners,
> *Coping with Executive Stress.*

Some of us can exercise, meditate, or do yoga or the relaxation exercises regularly and faithfully for months and months and still have trouble managing stress. But, there are alternatives for those persons and others who cannot handle stress on their own. We are referring here to help from others—psychologists, psychiatrists, or other counselors trained to help those with especially truculent stress problems.

James J. Lynch, professor and co-director of the Psycho-Physiology Laboratories at the University of Maryland

School of Medicine, has pointed out one reason why some of us cannot deal with stress on our own. Most adult stress, according to Professor Lynch, "has to do with interpersonal relationships, particularly those during childhood. In other words, we are not so much 'victims' of stress, as victims of our own personalities and conflicts."[1]

Dealing with personality and conflict problems is not something to be taken lightly. But, using the services of a trained professional to help you combat stress does not necessarily mean you'll have to spend years and years on the couch. Many persons find that they need to consult a therapist only during times of acute stress. It is not uncommon for someone to meet with a therapist or other counselor only about a dozen times. That counseling then helps get the person through the difficult period and also gives him the wherewithal to deal with any acute stressful periods in the future.

There are innumerable kinds of professional counseling techniques. If you think you need counseling to deal with stress, but are at a loss as to what type to choose, try asking for advice from your physician or a close friend or relative. Remember: There is no stigma attached today in undergoing psychological counseling. Seeing a counselor doesn't mean you're "crazy." On the contrary, it shows you know what you're doing; it shows you've recognized that you have a problem and are working with a trained expert to help solve that problem.

Here are brief descriptions of several types of counseling that have proven successful in helping people deal with stress.

Hypnosis

Earlier in chapter 6, we spent some time explaining how to do a series of relaxation exercises. The technique used in those exercises is known as autosuggestion, progressive relaxation, autogenic training, or self-hypnosis. During the relaxation exercises, you bring yourself into a deep psychological and physical state of total relaxation. This is very similar to what happens under hypnosis. Psychologists Robert L. Woolfolk and Frank C. Richardson, in fact, define hypnosis as "the altered state of consciousness that results from focusing awareness on a set of suggestions and allowing oneself to be receptive to those suggestions—all the while allowing free reign to one's powers of imagination."[2]

Doctors trained in hypnosis have used the technique to help patients get through many different types of medical procedures, including childbirth and dental work. In addition, hypnosis has been used successfully to cure persons of drug abuse, smoking, alcoholism, and insomnia, as well as many different types of psychological problems, including the inability to deal with stress, fear of flying, and the fear of public speaking (stage fright).

Hypnosis helps alleviate stress-related problems because—like meditation, progressive relaxation and yoga—hypnosis gets your mind and body to relax totally. Under hypnosis, muscle tension and fatigue eases, the heart slows down, and brain activity relaxes. When you are in a relaxed, hypnotic state, you are susceptible to suggestions that help you bring back your relaxed state after you come out of hypnosis. In this way, you can fight tension and anxiety by relaxing your body and mind totally any time you feel the need to do so. You will therefore be less prone to the destructive effects of stress.

"While hypnotized, you can reaffirm and reinforce a commitment to change both beliefs and behavior," note Woolfolk and Richardson. "When you are hypnotized, you are more receptive to suggestions you wish to follow. Thus, it is possible to use the hypnotic state as an opportunity to reprogram your mental computer in desired directions."[3]

You have to *want* to be hypnotized in order to benefit from it. This means that you should go into a hypnotic session with an open and receptive mind. You must take the attitude that you are going to cooperate and work with your hypnotist in order to help yourself deal with stress. Once you've been hypnotized a number of times, and feel the positive effects, you may want to learn techniques of self-hypnosis or autosuggestion so that you can bring on the hypnotic state at will.

Remember: Only seek help from a qualified practitioner of hypnosis. If you have any doubts, consult your physician.

Biofeedback

Another type of professional help that has proven effective in helping ease stress-related tension is biofeedback—the process by which the body regulates itself with the help of electronic monitoring equipment. Although the concept of biofeedback has been known for decades, it has only been in the last 15 years that the technique has been used widely therapeutically.

Today's biofeedback theory owes a good deal to the work of Dr. Hans Berger who, in the late 1920s, discovered the existence of brain waves and the relationship between specific brain wave patterns and mental states. Dr. Berger was the first to discover that when people close their eyes and relax, the pattern of electroencephalographic (EEG) waves emanating from their brains differs from the EEG pattern emitted when they have their eyes open. It was thus shown that EEG patterns are a mirror of our levels of tension and anxiety.

Since the time of Dr. Berger's experiments, researchers have uncovered four basic brain wave patterns. The different patterns show up when we are anxious (the beta pattern), relaxed (alpha), deep in thought (theta), and asleep (delta). The key to using biofeedback to fight stress is finding the alpha wave pattern. Biofeedback expert Barbara B. Brown explains: "The fact that, *in general,* the presence of alpha activity in the EEG and the absence of beta activity indicates a mental-emotional state of relaxed wakefulness is almost reason enough to suggest its use in individuals who complain of anxiety and whose EEG shows an abnormally low content of alpha."[4]

Psychologist Joseph Kamiya, a sleep researcher at the University of Chicago, was the first to discover that we can control our alpha brain wave patterns. In the early 1950s, Dr. Kamiya had sleep research volunteers ring bells when they thought they were emitting alpha waves. When he checked the bell ringing with the actual pattern of brain waves, Dr. Kamiya found that his subjects not only identified their own alpha states, but could start and stop them at will.

The next big breakthrough in biofeedback research came in the 1960s. Dr. Neal E. Miller, a professor of physiological psychology, and his associates at Rockefeller University succeeded in training rats to control their interior functions, such as heart rates and blood pressure. By 1966, Dr. Bernard Engle, a psychologist then working at the University of California, San Francisco, was reporting success in teaching volunteers to regulate their own heartbeats using biofeedback techniques. Today, biofeedback is used to control brain wave patterns, heartbeats, blood pressure, and even muscle tension.

There are many different types of biofeedback equipment in use today. But they all operate on the same basic principle: They teach a patient to control the changes taking place in the body by providing a display (either sight or sound) of the bodily changes.

The galvanic skin response (GSR) machine detects changes

in electrical activity at skin level and converts the activity into audible tones. Psychologists use GSR machines on patients who have trouble controlling tension and anxiety. When you become overly anxious or frightened, your nervous system sends impulses to the sweat glands and you begin to perspire. This is true at all times, even though the perspiration may not always be visible. When you perspire, the skin's resistance to electrical currents is reduced. And if you are hooked up to a GSR machine, the machine's tone will rise higher and higher the more anxious you get. Conversely, as you calm down, the tone lowers.

So, it's easy to see how you can use a GSR machine to control anxiety. You try to lower the machine's pitch, and if you do so, you are automatically lowering your anxiety level. No matter how you do it, you in effect teach yourself how to calm down during periods of stress. Once you've taught yourself to calm down using the GSR machine, you can apply what you've learned the next time you feel anxious in real life.

You usually hook into the machine with two electrodes taped to your fingers. You feel no electricity, no shock, and no burning sensation. There is nothing inserted into your skin. When the biofeedback instructor turns on the GSR, a very slight electrical current is sent through your skin. GSR equipment is sometimes part of so-called lie detector equipment. The idea is that you become anxious when you lie, and the machine can read the anxiety—not the lying. Some stripped-down GSR models are sold in electronic stores. If you buy one, you should be able to teach yourself how to use it fairly easily.

The electromyograph (EMG) biofeedback machine responds to movements in the muscles. It is used most often with patients who need to lower their blood pressure. But EMG machines also are used to help cure muscle spasms, insomnia, tension headaches, and facial tics.

The EMG measures things such as the blinking of an eyelid, the tightening of a bicep, or any other type of muscle-fiber contraction. The measurement takes place through metal electrodes taped on the body—on the forehead, for example, to deal with headaches—that pick up the bioelectrical currents given off when muscles contract. The signal is amplified a million times and is depicted on the EMG machine as a ticking noise that gets louder as the muscles contract, and quiets down as the muscles relax. It's kind of like a Geiger counter.

The EMG has proven to be most effective in relieving tension headaches caused by chronic tension in the scalp and neck muscles. With electrodes attached to the forehead to detect tension in the frontalis muscles, the patient tries to relax this area of the head. You know when you've successfully relaxed the frontalis because the EMG stops ticking. Some people successfully relax the muscles simply by repeating to themselves in an autosuggestive manner, "My forehead is relaxed; my forehead is relaxed; my forehead is *completely* relaxed." Others visualize themselves totally relaxed on a beach surrounded by calm water and a clear, blue sky. Others imagine themselves flying freely and easily on a supple magic carpet, soaring above the clouds in a totally relaxed environment.

Whatever visualization or autosuggestion technique you use, you will hear the evidence to help you learn to relax the frontalis. After working with the frontalis, you can work on relaxing other headache-causing muscles in the scalp, neck, and upper body.

Another biofeedback tool is the biofeedback thermometer, which is used to teach subjects to control their bodily temperature. Researchers have uncovered evidence indicating that if you can learn to increase the warmth in your hand, you will at the same time automatically increase the temperature in your head. By increasing the temperature in your head, you change the blood pressure and ease tension in your skull. This is why the hand-warming technique can help ease the pain of migraine headaches. Even though we still do not know the exact cause of migraines, it is believed that the pain comes from increased pressure in the blood vessels of the scalp caused by an increased flow of blood in the head.

Here's how the technique can work to prevent migraines. With one electrode placed in the middle of the right hand, and the other on the forehead, the patient tries to imagine his hand warming up. Some people picture themselves sitting in bright sunlight; others think of taking a bath in hot water. As the patient envisions the hand warming up, she is also looking at a dial on the extra-large biofeedback thermometer. You know your technique is working when you see the needle move toward the right. No one knows exactly why this works, but many people have reported that after learning to use the hand-warming technique with a biofeedback thermometer their migraines have decreased in both frequency and intensity.

One final basic type of biofeedback equipment, the EEG machine, measures alpha wave patterns. Brain waves are measured by the number of cycles they generate per second. The slowest patterns, delta waves, are emitted when you are in deep, dreamless sleep. The next fastest, the theta waves, come when you are either in a semiconscious state of drowsiness or in the dream portion of sleep, or during hallucinations or bursts of creativity. Next come the alpha waves, which usually come in bursts. Closing your eyes, for example, will increase the production of alpha waves by 15–20 percent. Beta waves are the fastest of all, and come when we are concentrating heavily or are under tension.

EEG biofeedback training helps you relax your mind, body, and nervous system. With a small sensor taped to your scalp, your brain waves are converted either into a visual or aural display, depending on the type of machine used. You set the machine for an alpha wave readout, so that it emits a loud clicking noise, say, when you are showing a strong, constant alpha wave pattern. The idea is to control your mind so that you are relaxed. As you do so, you'll be able to monitor the alpha wave pattern.

Stress Management Programs

At last count, there were about 120 of them. They have names like the Stress Institute, the Stress Control Center, the Center for Stress-Related Disorders, and Corporate Stress Control Services. They are businesses set up solely to offer stress management programs to individuals, as well as to corporations for their employees. There are also dozens of other institutes, spas, and other health-related organizations that offer special stress management counseling programs. Some large corporations even have their own stress clinics for employees.

Most of the techniques used in these specialized stress management programs already have been outlined in this book. These include meditation, exercise, biofeedback, hypnosis, psychological counseling, and diet and nutrition advice. Some of these stress control programs are very expensive. The Menninger Foundation in Topeka, Kansas, for example, runs a program for executives with a price tag of $2,300. It is not uncommon for other stress clinics to charge about $1,500 per person per week.

The stress management field has its share of unscrupulous entrepreneurs and charlatans who charge large fees to teach unproven or unworkable stress management techniques. Said Paul Rosch, president of the American Institute of Stress: "If anybody says they're going to give you a stress reduction program in a day, forget it. It's a scam."[5]

Most legitimate stress control concerns offer individualized stress management advice to each client. To begin with, the client is interviewed extensively and given a series of tests such as the Holmes-Raye Life Events Chart. Then an individualized program is drawn up that typically includes instruction in relaxation and exercise programs, advice on diet and nutrition, and a consultation with a clinical psychologist or other trained therapist.

Psychodrama and "Shock Spot" Stress Control

There are so many different types of psychological counseling available that it would be fruitless even to give a capsule description of each one. Suffice it to say that nearly all of the different types of counseling have proven successful in fighting stress-related tension. This includes the traditional patient-on-the-couch individual session with a psychiatrist, as well as the many different and varied types of group therapies.

One type of group therapy, psychodrama, has several techniques designed especially to work with stress. Psychodrama is a discipline pioneered by Dr. J. L. Moreno in the 1920s. It uses dramatic enactment in a group setting to help you gain insight into your problems. Psychodrama is especially useful for helping people understand how they react to stressful situations because during the psychodrama you recreate stressful incidents from the past and use action techniques including role reversal to combat stress problems.

One psychodrama exercise uses the "shock spot" theory to work with stress. It begins with a group of about 20 participants filling out the Holmes and Raye chart (see pp. 4–9). Then the group is divided into three subgroups based on the scores they compiled. One group brings together all those who scored in the mild risk category. One group is composed of those with scores in the moderate risk category, and the final group is made up of those individuals whose totals indicated that they run a major risk of developing a stress-related illness.

After the subgroups are chosen, the psychodrama leader asks each group collectively to come up with a list of things they do to help cope with stress. Each group is given 15 minutes to do so. Then, a spokesperson from each group reads the list aloud. The psychodrama leader then comments on the different styles of coping.

Each member of each group is then asked to list all the people, things, or events he interacts with on a daily basis. Participants are asked to be expansive and creative in drawing up this list. Each group member then reads aloud his list of persons, places, and things that cause tension. The participants are then asked to look over their lists and figure out which stressor causes them the most trouble. Then the "drama" part of the psychodrama comes into play.

Participants are asked to take on a posture, gesture, and verbalization that they think best describes their worst stress, and interact with all the members of the group. The leader encourages the members to be as expressive as they can be. For example, one person begins shouting, screaming, and bumping around the room imitating the dirty, noisy bus she must take to and from work every morning. She mills through the group, making sure she interacts with all the others.

After all the participants have had the chance to act out their stressors, the leaders ask each one to select the one group member he was able to relate to best during the "milling about" phase. After all, the members are paired off, the leaders ask the pairs to sit facing one another.

The leader then explains the shock-spot theory; each of us has his own bodily "shock spot"—maybe a nervous stomach, tense neck muscles, chest pains, tension headaches, diarrhea, or whatever—which responds when we're under stress. Each participant is asked to think about the one bodily part that is most affected by stress.

Now some more drama comes into play. One at a time, the pairs begin to help each other by taking on the role of their own shock spots and describing what it is that the shock spot does. In each pair, the person in the role of the shock spot talks to the other person, who nonverbally acknowledges the feelings of his partner. Then the pairs switch roles, but this time, the feelings of the shock spot *are* acknowledged verbally. The dialogue can be ended at any time by the person whose problem is being dealt with.

After each pair has a chance to act out their shock spots, the group as a whole discusses how they felt as they acted out their problem areas. The individual can now identify shock spots, confront his feelings around the shock spot, and develop insight into the causes of the shock spot. Once you identify and talk about your shock spot, you can then begin to control it.

Another psychodrama method for dealing with stress is to have each member of the group draw up a list of the people—individuals, family members, co-workers, or anyone else—that he seeks support from in times of need. The things to keep in mind are: who the most important person in your support network is, how you support yourself during stressful periods, who, if anyone, is missing from your supporters, and if there has been any major change in the group in the previous year.

Then, in the drama portion, each person in turn selects group members to represent each supporter on his list, and asks each person to take a posture, gesture, or phrase that best sums up the essence of that support. Someone representing a mother, for example, might be asked to stand protectively near the person with her arms outstretched, or a person representing a religious counselor might stand far away with his hands prayerfully clasped.

First the leader asks the person and his dramatized supporters to strike up a dialogue. Then, a role reversal takes place, and the supporter says what he appreciates most about the person.

The shock spot and supporter techniques act as ways in which each person in the group can get insights into behavior patterns he may not ever have thought through fully. By dramatizing their problems, the psychodrama can awaken the participants to the things they can do in their everyday life to combat stress.

Adopting a Code of Behavior

This final section contains what could be both the easiest and most difficult advice to follow in this book. We are referring here to Dr. Selye's solution to controlling the harmful effects of stress: adopting a "code of behavior," a ready-made framework for dealing with the events in your life to maximize happiness and minimize tension, anxiety, and stress. The easy part is promising yourself that you'll adopt such a code. The hard part is actually changing your life and putting the code into action.

Here are some hints borrowed from Dr. Selye's book, *Stress Without Distress*. The key to a code of behavior designed to give you peace of mind and fulfillment is to strike a balance in your life between meaningful work and relaxation. Your work must give you satisfaction. It must have attainable goals and it must be in a field you respect— either in business, art, science, or whatever.

Your code of behavior, Dr. Selye claims, should also strike a balance between doing things for yourself and doing things for others. The primary object is to gain as much goodwill through your work as possible, and to expand your network of friends.

Here are some ways to help you along this admirable path.

• Don't be a perfectionist, because perfection is impossible. If you strive for perfection, you invite continual disappointment.

• Strive for simplicity. It's much easier to cope with the vicissitudes of life if you avoid burdening yourself with unnecessary complications.

• Always question whether your problems are really worth fighting for. If you think through each problematic situation in life, you'll probably find that some things in which you've invested a good deal of stress, tension, and anxiety, may mean very little to you.

• Don't neglect the power of positive thinking. Dwelling on the negative, ugly, and painful is self-defeating and brings too much stress. Accentuate the positive, even when you've "failed" at something.

• Don't procrastinate, especially when undertaking unpleasant tasks. It's usually best to dive right in and get them over with, rather than waiting and building up more anxiety than is needed.

• Remember that not everyone is going to wind up on top in all situations. There will be many more losers than winners in life, many more followers than leaders. It's simply the natural order of things. So don't let the lack of success gnaw at you. As long as you give it your best, if you fail to reach a goal totally, it is no cause for feeling sorry for yourself.

• Finally, remember that all of us are different, and that what works for others will not necessarily work for you. That is why each of us needs our own code of behavior. We need to stick with it through the good and bad times. Having such a code is sure to minimize the harmful effects of stress.

1. James J. Lynch, writing in *The Washington Post,* Book World, October 17, 1982, p. 11.
2. Robert L. Woolfolk and Frank C. Richardson, *Stress, Sanity and Survival* (New York: New American Library, 1978), p.157.
3. Woolfolk and Richardson, *Survival,* p. 159.
4. Barbara B. Brown, *Stress and the Art of Biofeedback* (New York: Bantam Books, 1978), p. 185.
5. Paul Rosch, quoted in the *Wall Street Journal,* September 30, 1982.

Bibliography

ANDERSON, BOB. *Stretching*. Shelter Publications, 1980.

BENNETT, WILLIAM, and GURIN, JOEL. *The Dieter's Dilemma*. New York: Basic Books, Inc., Publishers, 1982.

BENSON, HERBERT. *The Relaxation Response*. New York: William Morrow & Co., Inc., 1975.

"Biofeedback in Action." *Medical World News*, March 3, 1979.

BROWN, BARBARA B. *Stress and the Art of Biofeedback*. New York: Bantam Books, 1977.

CARRINGTON, PATRICIA et al. "The Use of Meditation: Relaxation Techniques for the Management of Stress in a Working Population." *Journal of Occupational Medicine*, April 1980.

COLEMAN, VERNON. *Stress Control*. Transatlantic, 1979.

COOPER, KENNETH H. *Aerobics*. New York: Bantam Books, 1969.

COOPER, MILDRED, and COOPER, KENNETH H. *Aerobics for Women*. New York: Bantam Books, 1972.

"Dealing With Troubled Sleep." *Business Week*, October 11, 1982.

DEVANANDA, SWAMI VISHNU. *Meditation and Mantras*. OM Lotus Publishing, 1978.

Bibliography

DOUGLASS, MERRILL E. "Stress and Personal Performance." *The Personnel Administrator,* August 1977.

Executive Health Examiners. *Coping With Executive Stress.* New York: McGraw-Hill Book Company, 1982.

FENVES, STEVEN J. et al. *Stress: A Reference Manual.* Cambridge, Mass.: The MIT Press, 1965.

FIXX, JAMES. *The Complete Book of Running.* New York: Random House, Inc., 1978.

FRIEDMAN, MEYER, and ROSENMAN, RAY H. *Type A Behavior and Your Heart.* New York: Fawcett, Crest, 1974.

GOLDBERG, PHILIP. *Executive Health.* New York: McGraw-Hill Book Company, 1978.

GORMAN, TRISHA. "Women and Heart Disease." *Working Woman,* September 1982.

GUENTHER, ROBERT. "Stress Management Plans Abound, But Not All Programs are Well Run." *The Wall Street Journal,* September 30, 1982.

KRAMER, ANN, ed. *Woman's Body: An Owner's Manual.* The Diagram Group, 1977.

LAMOTT, KENNETH. *Escape from Stress.* New York: Berkley Books, 1976.

LEVINSON, HARRY. *Executive Stress.* New York: Harper & Row, Publishers, 1966.

MADDERS, JANE. *Stress and Relaxation.* New York: Arco Publishing Co., Inc., 1979.

MATTESON, MICHAEL T. and ICANCEVICH, JOHN M. *Managing Job Stress and Health.* New York: The Free Press, 1982.

MCGUIGAN, F. J. et al., eds. *Stress and Tension Control.* New York: Plenum Publishing Corporation, 1980.

MCQUADE, WALTER, and AIKMAN, ANN. *Stress.* New York: Bantam Books, 1975.

MENDELSON, WALLACE B. et al. *Human Sleep and its Disorders.* Plenum Publishing Corporation, 1977.

MORSE, DONALD ROY, and FURST, M. LAWRENCE *Stress for*

Success. New York: Van Nostrand Reinhold Company, 1979.

PELLETIER, KENNETH R. *Mind as Healer, Mind as Slayer: A Holistic Approach to Preventing Stress Disorders.* Delta, 1977.

SATCHIDANANDA, YOGIRAJ SRI SWAMI. *Integral Yoga Hatha.* New York: Holt, Reinhart and Winston, 1970.

"Secret of Coping With Stress: Interview With Dr. Hans Selye." *U.S. News & World Report,* March 21, 1977.

SEHNART, KEITH W. *Stress/Unstress.* Augsburg Publishing, 1981.

SELIGER, SUSAN. "Stress Can Be Good for You." *New York,* August 2, 1982.

SELYE, HANS. *Stress Without Distress.* Signet, 1974.

———. *The Stress of Life.* rev. ed. McGraw-Hill Book Company, 1978.

STROEBEL, CHARLES F. *The Quieting Reflex.* New York: G. P. Putnam's Sons, 1982.

TAVERNIER, GERARD. "The High Cost and Stress of Relocation." *Management Review,* July 1980.

WHEATLEY, DAVID, ed. *Stress and the Heart.* 2d ed. Raven, 1981.

WOOLFOLK, ROBERT L., and RICHARDSON, FRANK C. *Stress, Sanity and Survival.* New York: New American Library, 1978.

YATES, JERE E. *Managing Stress.* New York: AMACOM, 1979.

ABOUT THE AUTHOR

Marc Leepson has written numerous articles on health, exercise, and nutrition. His work has been published in *The New York Times, Washington Post, Chicago Tribune,* and *Smithsonian Magazine,* among others. He is author of EXECUTIVE FITNESS (McGraw-Hill, 1982).

A Vietnam veteran, Mr. Leepson, now 39, has practiced many of the stress-reduction techniques covered in his book. He is currently staff writer with Editorial Research Reports, a news service published by Congressional Quarterly in Washington, D.C.

How's Your Health?

Bantam publishes a line of informative books, written by top experts to help you toward a healthier and happier life.